Partnership Working

Anthony Douglas

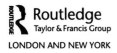

Routledge
Taylor & Francis Group

LONDON AND NEW YORK

First published 2009
by Routledge
2 Park Square, Milton Park, Abingdon, Oxon OX14 4RN

Simultaneously published in the USA and Canada
by Routledge
711 Third Avenue, New York, NY 10017

*Routledge is an imprint of the Taylor & Francis Group, an informa
business*

Typeset in Galliard by
HWA Text and Data Management, London

British Library Cataloguing in Publication Data
A catalogue record for this book is available from the British Library

Library of Congress Cataloging-in-Publication Data

Douglas, Anthony, 1949-
   Partnership working / Anthony Douglas
        p. cm.
   1. Social service—Great Britain. 2. Partnership—Great Britain.
3. Private-sector cooperation. 4. Community-based social services—
Great Britain. I. Title.
   HV245.D685 2008
   361.941—dc22   2008023491

ISBN10: 0–415–31165–9 (hbk)
ISBN10: 0–415–31166–7 (pbk)
ISBN10: 0–203–46278–5 (pbk)

ISBN13: 978–0–415–31165–6 (hbk)
ISBN13: 978–0–415–31166–3 (pbk)
ISBN13: 978–0–203–46278–2 (pbk)

Partnership Working

Partnership working is recognised as a crucial means of improving social care services, and is a non-negotiable part of the government's intention to provide a seamless care service. However, for everyone involved in partnership working, the question is: how can it be carried out successful in practice?

This book is both an introduction and an in-depth analysis of partnership working across the public sector in the UK. In a comprehensive discussion Anthony Douglas explores:

- the history of partnership working, its theoretical base and practical applications
- why partnership working is important
- how professionals are already working together
- how to develop good relationships and address common difficulties
- how to ensure that partnership working really does result in better practice
- the future of partnership working.

The analysis and examples range across the whole of the public sector with a primary focus on social care. Drawing on up-to-date research and using plenty of practical examples and thinking points, *Partnership Working* will be of interest to students, researchers and policy makers at all levels, and practitioners and managers of front-line services.

Anthony Douglas is Chief Executive of the Children and Family Court Advisory and Support Service (Cafcass), Chair of the British Association for Adoption and Fostering (BAAF) and a visiting fellow of the University of East Anglia. He has written three previous books on social care. He was awarded a CBE in 2008 for services to family justice and adoption.

To the many people who use services and the many staff who care about them, who I have had the privilege of working with and learning from during the last 33 years

Contents

Figures

Combination carries strength with it. It's dreadful to adversaries.
(Oliver Cromwell)

'We will always be here, trying to make shattered lives worth living: partnership with Halesowen College for basic tuition, courses and added life chances for victim survivors'.
(Halesowen Women's Refuge mission statement)

Without teamwork, you're dead.
(Terry Green, ex fire-fighter)

He travels in mid-river always.
(Michael Ondaatje, *Anil's Ghost*)

Preface

My book is about partnership working in general and social care in particular. It seeks to answer basic questions about partnership working which I have heard from students and government ministers alike: why, who, what for, how, when and where? Partnership working is an idea whose time has arrived ahead of the cavalry – my book attempts in a small way to reduce the waiting time.

I hope my book can be read from cover to cover – every author's aspiration of course – and also that it can be dipped into at any point. I would like you as a reader to find something of interest in each section, especially a practical application.

Throughout my book, I have sought to showcase partnership working at its best. Just as Leonardo Da Vinci's machines were ahead of his time, including designs for helicopters and hang gliders that could not fly because other required materials and technologies had not yet been invented, partnership working pioneers often lack support for their radical schemes. This book is also for them.

I have tried to convey how much positive good can come from partnership working. If I have also conveyed doubt, it is because partnership working is difficult despite its apparent simplicity. If it goes wrong, the consequences can be serious or fatal. If it is not too grandiose an aim, I would like my book to play a part in promoting successful partnership working, and to reduce the risk of it disintegrating in any one case or service, to the detriment of all involved.

Anthony Douglas
London and Suffolk, 2008

1 A rationale for partnership working

Key messages

- Partnership working is likely to be a major public sector paradigm for the next 25 years
- Partnership working can be an inspirational framework for people who use services and professionals alike
- Partnership working is not a magic solution for complex social care problems
- Despite its ubiquity, partnership working can leave participants confused about its purpose and unclear about their role, without clear leadership, guidance and support
- At the end of the day, partnership working is the only public policy show in town which has the potential to successfully address the big issues of our times such as social exclusion

---

First, the definition

The P word

Partnership working is a key twenty-first century concept with multiple meanings yet still with no commonly understood definition. 'The quiet revolution of joined-up working', conveys the way in which partnership working is now obligatory throughout the public sector, more through expectation than a set of legal requirements (Crawford 1997). Partnership working has become 'the main vehicle for policy implementation across a broad range of activities' (Balloch and Taylor 2001). Every new government strategy, from animal health and welfare to road safety, majors on the P word. The vast majority of new services or projects, whichever level of government starts them, or whichever the sector, will include one or more partnerships. Partnership working is non-negotiable without that being explicit. In social care, Joint Area Review (JAR) recommendations are always made to a council 'and its partners', highlighting their joint responsibility and accountability. A similar framework will be used in new Comprehensive Area Assessments from April 2009. The requirement to work together is now written into virtually every new policy, procedure, job description and person profile throughout social care. For example, 'Understand what "multi-agency working" means for you and your work environment' is a key section of the Children's Workforce Development Council's Induction Standards for all professionals working with children young people and their families (CWDC 2006).

The public sector is packed with consortia, shared services, collaborations, trusts, merging organisations, voluntary shared membership agreements, coalitions of organisations forming to campaign on specific issues, and mutual assistance programmes. However, like Plato's forms, partnership is a theoretical concept which is often over-simplified in the manner of Woody Allen, when he was asked what Tolstoy's *War and Peace* was about and replied, 'it's a story about Russia'. Many of the new organisational arrangements for partnerships are becoming as complex as the social problems they have been set up to solve. In other words, they have the potential to become 'the undefinable in pursuit of the unachievable' (Powell and Dowling 2006).

The more complex it is, the more likely it is to need a partnership

Having said that, partnership working is not – and should never be – a service or an end in itself. It is a process and a mindset, one outcome of which may be a better service. Its relevance to and prevalence in social care lies in the complex nature of social care problems, which usually require the input of many people and agencies working effectively together. As Peter Beresford has said, 'Social care is not rocket science. It is much more complex and subtle than that' (Beresford 2005).

The expectation of partnership holds true at every level. Each social care case will involve a partnership between professionals and one or more people who use services. Today's social worker or care manager is part advocate, part safeguarder and part resource controller. She or he will have to discuss an individual service user's needs with many other people, all of whom may have their own perspective to add. For example, to set up the smallest care package, a care manager may still need to talk to the contracts team, finance team and brokerage team inside their agency.

The outcomes of a single social care intervention can be stunning. T, a child from Malaysia, in the English care system and unable to return home, was able to be placed with good family carers in the Philippines due to the flair and diligence of a manager in The Adolescent and Children's Trust (TACT) and a social worker in a West Midlands Council. These two professionals worked together for months to achieve a successful outcome for that child. In another example of partnership working which improves lives, two single parents, each with an eight-year-old child, share a house and jointly foster a child. A teacher who also lives in the house shares in the child's care, as does the child's mother who visits from time to time. Shared care has moved from the margin to the mainstream in many families, and families in the care system are no exception.

In fact, the only way in which the state can ensure that more than one million vulnerable children and adults in the UK every year receive enough support, is by mobilising the wider UK population to become involved: as professional staff, as informal carers, as formal carers – and by promoting a stronger sense of society and collective responsibility. Margaret Thatcher's famous phrase, 'there is no such thing as society' holds true in as much as the homogenous 'traditional' society in the UK has largely disappeared – witness the decline in membership of social institutions like political parties. But this rallying cry to the small-minded ignored the existence of new organisations and communities within the UK, many of which have grown in strength and purpose in the intervening years, like social networks and some churches, whose membership is increasing as a consequence of the search by citizens for meaning in life.

'Working together' : as close to a definition as it gets

No two words convey the essence of partnership working as clearly as 'working together'. The words are simple to say yet much harder to do.

Working Together, originally the title of Government child protection guidance (DH, Home Office, DfEE 1999), and the headline phrase in many government initiatives since, has come to mean:

- Effective communication and action between practitioners, and/or between practitioners and people who use services plus their families and carers to achieve a common goal.
- The development of structures and systems such as case conferences, case reviews, core groups, strategy meetings and information-sharing protocols, all of which are intended to deliver better outcomes.
- Close and effective collaboration between agency managers facing a common problem, collaboration which can take a number of forms, such as a joint service managed by one partner agency on behalf of both.
- A particular focus on the reduction of harm, or the risk of harm, or the promotion of health and well-being.

Stating the obvious, *working together* means not working in isolation from other professionals and people who use services. It means always working as part of a team: partnership is essentially teamwork with a fancy name. As the then chairman Lord Sainsbury said to a group of trainee managers in Sainsbury's, one of whom is now a social care manager I know, 'You're a team. TEAM equals Together Everyone Achieves More'. Being able as an individual to work as a member of a number of teams simultaneously is a pre-requisite of effective partnership working. To paraphrase Norman O.

Working together, supporting together

On a visit to a local Cafcass team, whilst waiting for a team meeting to start, a practitioner came up to me and said, 'Nice to see you again. Do you remember me?' After naming various places I had worked, to each of which he said "fraid not', I said, 'I'm really sorry, I give up', to which he replied, 'You were my social worker'. He had been one of my first cases. I had helped him, his brothers and his mum. They were children in need, and young carers some of the time. 'You took an interest in us' he said, 'and took us to a Spurs game, then for something to eat'. Being an Arsenal season ticket holder, this clearly went beyond the call of duty! I am not sure how many times I visited the family to offer help, but it was probably not that many. The meaning of the story is that for some people who are vulnerable or isolated, to feel respected and supported by somebody means a lot, even if that professional feels that they have not been able to do much at all.

Brown, professional polygamy is not just desirable, it is essential (Brown 1990). Having said that, teams are only performance-enhancing up to a point. It is individuals who provide the bulk of social care services, and they do this whether or not they work in teams. It is the relationship between the individual practitioner and the individual service user that lies at the heart of social care services (see Chapter 3).

Partnership working lies behind most great achievements. The political philosopher John Rawls said that individual achievement is a myth and any individual success is due to the efforts of many others and of society as a whole by supporting, helping and providing resources to that individual (quoted in Bateman 2006).

Partnership terminology – some definitions from the field

The endless variations in the definition of partnership working can be illustrated by the overlapping terms used within drugs work (National Treatment Agency 2005).

* *Partnership work*: can be defined as organisations with differing goals and traditions, yet needing to work together (Home Office 1992).
* *Joint working*: involves drug services developing working relationships with other drug-related organisations or services to 'help establish the broadest range of seamless service delivery' (National Treatment Agency 2002).
* *Shared care*: the joint participation of specialists and primary care practitioners, especially GPs and pharmacists, in the planned delivery of

care for patients with a drug misuse problem, 'informed by an enhanced information exchange beyond routine discharge and referral letters' (Department of Health, 1995).

• *Integrated care*: an approach that 'seeks to combine and co-ordinate all the services required to meet the assessed needs of an individual' (Effective Interventions Unit 2002).

Moving the goalposts – by widening them

Voluntary organisations have traditionally been creative and progressive, delivering demonstration projects for newly identified needs. Often, the small projects and partnerships they set up to meet these needs go onto become mainstream services. One example is the research partnership between Save the Children and Women's Aid which resulted in the publication of *Safe Learning*, the first resource guide about the social and educational needs of children and young people affected by domestic violence (Mill and Church 2006). The broader focus of this individual research partnership has helped professional staff across agencies build up a stronger knowledge base about the needs of children and young people facing these pressures, and through that to make more rounded assessments of the needs of children growing up in households with domestic violence. These wider considerations now form the basis of routine assessments for children in private law cases under the Adoption and Children Act 2002 and the Children and Adoption Act 2006. In this sense, one of the core functions of partnership working is to add to the knowledge base about a social issue with several dimensions, and to seek to widen the remit of statutory agencies to take into account those dimensions.

'I can swim but not yet': a parable about partnership working

A Director of Children's Services, visiting a primary school, sat down to talk with a five-year-old girl. She was proud and enthusiastic about what she could do. She said 'I can draw. I can get my own breakfast. I know the way to school. I can swim. I can read big books'. The list went on. The director congratulated her, then moved on to speak with the boy next to her. After a short while, the girl tapped him on the arm and said to him with a thoughtful expression, 'You know I said I can swim? Well I can, but not yet.'

Vague or loose descriptors for partnership working need to be made as specific and detailed as possible, to avoid misunderstandings between professionals, or with people who use services, about what will actually happen in practice. Expectations of partnership working can easily translate into expectations of joint services which may never materialise.

Working together, joint working, or partnership working – the terms are for practical purposes interchangeable – are the heart and soul of modern social care services. They stand for a civilised and civilising relationship between a state and its citizens.

Some urgent reasons for partnership working

The need for collaborative advantage

Without a compelling set of reasons to start and persevere with a partnership, it will probably fail, given the other competing priorities and constant pressure those at the heart of every partnership face. It must add value and convey 'collaborative advantage' that offers more than any one person or agency can achieve by themselves (Huxham and Vangen 2005). Generally speaking, if the need for partnership working is staring you in the face, go for it. If it isn't, be very careful. Don't be seduced by the rhetoric. This rule applies

---

Falling between stools

Steve is 33, single, out of work and depressed. He has no formal skills or qualifications. Several nights a week he gets drunk at a town centre pub, and then starts picking fights and assaulting women. He is often arrested but just as quickly released, and is on the edge of custody daily. Two psychiatric assessments concluded he is anti-social and vulnerable, but not mentally ill. He also falls outside adult social care services' eligibility criteria. The police are frustrated that, as they see it, no agency is 'doing anything'. A residents' action group complains to the local newspaper in a similar vein.

Convening an inter-agency review is important as Steve's needs may suddenly escalate to the point where he does warrant help. Effective communication between professionals is vital with someone like Steve who may pass through several 'revolving doors' in the course of a week. An incident log can help, maintained by a lead agency, in which every incident is reported so that a trend or sequence can be mapped and understood, perhaps before it is too late. Steve needs a 'lead professional' or care manager who receives all information about him, analyses what is happening and has the delegated authority to mobilise help when it is needed, which is likely to be during a crisis.

to seemingly straightforward joint working arrangements as well as major partnership programmes.

The single greatest, or main reason for partnership working is that no single professional social care worker or agency can by themselves and in isolation deliver significant social change for an individual, a social group or a community. To make a real difference to everyday social problems such as homelessness, child neglect, dementia care, or acute depression, it is very likely that more than one professional and more than one agency will need in every instance to work together effectively.

Social exclusion: where partnerships are most needed

Users of social care services tend to be disproportionately socially excluded. Some face a bleak and violent reality. A younger brother was assaulted by his older brother because if he went to work the family income from benefits would be cut. At an attendance centre in Bolton in 1998, a 14-year-old boy, already a father of two children, stripped off to reveal he was wearing a £450 bullet-proof vest. There was a contract out on his life. Inmates in Huntercombe, the young offenders institution (YOI) near Oxford, over-estimate the size of the prison population by a factor of up to 100, because the majority of people they know have been to prison (source: discussion with Graham Badman, Managing Director for Children's Services for Kent County Council and formerly Chief Education Officer for Oxfordshire).

Social exclusion is a firmly established cross-cutting issue which in recent times has defeated the efforts of every government to solve. Most social problems faced by individuals or social groups require a concerted and sustained effort by more than one agency to solve, and even then the problem may last for years or even centuries. In 1997, the incoming Labour government in the UK announced it intended to end child poverty by 2020, and by 2010 to halve the numbers of affected children. Depending on the measurement scales used, the UK is the fourth or fifth richest country in the world, yet we have the fourth largest proportion of children living in poverty in Europe, exceeded only by Poland, Hungary and Latvia. By 2008, the target remained a long way off. Admittedly, considerable progress has been made, and the government invested an extra £1,715 million in its 2008 budget, aiming to take a further 250,000 children out of poverty. It has also set up a Joint Child Poverty Unit across the two key government departments concerned – the Department for Children, Schools and Families (DCSF) and the Department for Work and Pensions (DWP), one of an increasing number of cross-governmental teams with a fresh remit for partnership working.

However, tackling centuries-old problems will take decades at the very least. East London has been poorer than west London for over 500 years, with little sign that underlying structural inequalities are being reduced. For example, a boy growing up in Muswell Hill can expect to live 5.5 years longer than a boy growing up in White Hart Lane, 2 miles away (London Borough

The victim and the aggressor

In my own work, I can define the incidents or events which changed my own professional mindset. One, in the 1980s, was when a father I was working with who had sexually abused his children, and had threatened to kill my family and myself, hung himself. It taught me that behind most aggression lies intense pain. That is not to excuse aggression, but in social care, the explanation for unacceptable behaviour has to be sought and found if vulnerable people are to be helped, or if their destructive behaviour is to be stopped.

of Haringey, 2005), and children from the five per cent most disadvantaged households in Kent are more than 50 times more likely to have multiple problems at age 30 than those from the top 50 per cent of households (Kent County Council). Children from poor families are 13 times more likely to have accidents than children from the highest social classes (The Child Accident Prevention Trust). The impact of poverty on a child needs to be taken into account, as do many other dimensions, when carrying out an assessment of need (Gill and Jack 2008).

Partnerships at every level are needed to begin to solve such deep-rooted problems and, in a positive sense, 'partnership has put excluded groups and communities onto the agenda in a way they have not been before' (Balloch and Taylor 2001). A start can be made by making it easier to access services in the first place. Too often, people needing help are sent off with an address and a phone number, which may or may not be right, and left to their own devices. It is no wonder that, having plucked up courage over a long period of time to ask for help, many give up in a split second, sensing hostility or indifference. A partnership agreement between local front-line agencies, with a signposting and 'referral-on' protocol, can help to ease people's anxieties about officialdom, even trendy contemporary officialdom, which can be just as daunting.

Shining a light on silo mentalities – and opening them up

Silo-working – defined as only being interested in your own agenda, and going your own way, whether as an individual or an organisation – has become a term of contempt and abuse. As Kathy Sutton said of the criminal justice system, it remains 'a cumbersome, outmoded system operating in silos, placing organisational concerns above those of the user' (Sutton 2005).

Silo mentalities are not confined to front line public services. They are a common phenomenon, reflecting what was an acceptable working practice until quite recently. Research studies looking at a mixture of organisational structures have noted widespread and chronic insularity. For instance, writing about university teaching cultures, Genn, Partington and Wheeler found that:

> the disciplinary-based structures of universities do not always provide ideal conditions for collaboration between lawyers and academics in other disciplines, with universities still reflecting a Victorian 'brigading' of knowledge. While there have been moves towards larger multi-disciplinary schools, these have often been driven by managerial rather than academic pressures. There is a need for active efforts on the part of funders and university administrators to promote cross-disciplinary collaboration.
>
> (Genn *et al.* 2006)

The lack of partnership working in practice, certainly compared to its rhetorical dominance, has also been identified in a plethora of inspection reports and serious case reviews and inquiries. However, innumerable organisations know what must be done to narrow the gap. As Helen Ghosh, Permanent Secretary at the Department for the Environment, Food and Rural Affairs in England (Defra) stated:

> The crucial change we have to make focuses on collaborative behaviour. The management board isn't made up of director generals with individual policy silos. Each has a portfolio of interests that will encourage a genuinely collaborative approach to making decisions and moving priorities around. It is this behavioural and cultural change for all of us in Defra which is the greatest challenge, because unless we get the behaviour right, then the structural reforms won't work.
>
> (Ghosh 2007)

The high stakes for partnership working in social care

The same is true – and probably more so – for social care, because social care decisions, especially those about personal liberty, are amongst the most serious the state has to make. Social care is literally a cradle to grave service, which travels the same journey as life itself, through from pre-birth cases where an individual mother can be addicted to drugs or alcohol and may already have caused damage to her unborn child, all the way through to the care of a terminally ill patient in the last phase of their life. Whilst many of us will receive the help we need from a single professional such as a GP, the persistent and enduring problems which form the average social care caseload will only be helped through a multi-agency or interdisciplinary approach. As Cameron and Masterson say in relation to older people: 'It is clear that no one profession can provide adequate care for an increasingly ageing population who are more likely to live longer with multiple pathologies' (Cameron and

The confused and Kafkaesque professional system: Olive and Peter's story

We have twin girls aged 5. Both have a moderate learning disability. One also has autism. We're totally confused with all the different professionals and agencies we have to deal with. The following are some of the people we see on a regular basis: GP, counselling nurse, speech and language therapist, occupational therapist, psychiatrist, psychologist, teacher, classroom assistant, ophthalmologist, audiologist and administrators. We're so confused sometimes. We don't understand the different roles and have so many appointments that clash. Can nobody or no system sort it out?

Others, unable to access services at all, may find Olive and Peter's dilemmas a little self-indulgent, in that despite having so much help, they still complain!

Parents 'Olive and Peter', quoted in *Developing a Model for Integrated Primary, Community and Continuing Care in the Midland Health Board (Ireland)*, Executive Summary, June 2003

Masterson 1998). The same holds true for children, young people and adults of working age who need social care support. The partnership working imperative confronts social care professionals daily.

The consequence of poor partnership working or poorly co-ordinated services can be devastating. Families with a disabled family member may have contact with ten or more professionals from different professions. Some case conferences have as many as 30 professionals present, presenting a massive co-ordination challenge to the lead professional, but mostly to families themselves (see Olive and Peter's story in the box).

Such co-ordination is routine in some fields. For example, it takes 37 people in an operating theatre to sew an arm back on, and the operation relies upon a high level of co-operation between a range of specialists, generalists and back-up staff. However, in the social care field, many people who use services and professionals continue to report poor communication within multi-agency services (Kirk and Glendinning 2004). Faced with this, 'families may often end up taking on the role of co-ordinator themselves' (Townsley *et al.* 2004). Integrated working can reduce professional duplication (see below).

The importance of whole-system partnership working

Whole-system partnership working means numerous functions and agencies are required to provide services to members of a particular service user

How Chris made life simpler for Jane

Chris is a support worker from the flexible support team in Kirby. Jane is a 13-year-old whose parents had separated, had poor attendance and who, following a bereavement, had begun self-harming. 'By completing a Common Assessment Framework (CAF), and getting a full picture of Jane's needs and the agencies working with her, we were able to provide services much more effectively', said Chris. 'Previously, she was in contact with eight people, which involved a lot of duplication of effort and was overwhelming for her. By understanding her needs better, we were able to reduce this to just three – with great results. She's much happier, is dealing with her grief and has returned to education, learning new vocational skills.'

Source: Department for Children, Schools and Families

group. All children in care require educational, social work and health service support, and many, in addition, will also need other forms of support such as specialist housing. People with a severe learning disability are likely to require specialist nursing, a GP, social care support, support for their carers and extra care housing. Whole-system partnerships will need to be able to mobilise other forms of help in particular situations for people who use services and who have extra needs. Mobilising whole systems effectively can usually only be done by a care manager or network manager with skills in partnership working.

The bigger picture

Social care problems need partnership solutions, and in this respect social care is part of a much bigger picture. The need for effective partnership action to tackle global problems has become increasingly apparent. For example, the number of eels in the North Sea is 90 per cent down in recent years. Eels take no notice of maritime boundaries, so collaboration between northern European countries is needed and underway to protect and replenish stocks. Two co-operatives in Coope Tarcoles, Costa Rica, developed a partnership for responsible fishing, which has improved environmental management, produced a more sustainable approach to fishing, and developed new fishing businesses to ensure knowledge transfer about responsible fishing to the next generation (FAO, Costa Rica 2006). Ten billion spam emails a day are sent within the European Union, costing 2.5 billion euros a year – a global anti-spam partnership is essential. Apart from the visits of 200 scientists and explorers a year, Antarctica is an uninhabited and uninhabitable continent the size of Europe, supported by 12 countries working in partnership as best as they can to protect its resources.

Some intergovernmental projects have proved too complex to deliver, like the European Rail Traffic Management System (ERTMS), which has been unable to bring different national operating practices into one single system. Every integration project has to be clear at the outset that it can succeed, and what help it needs to be able to do so (see Chapter 5).

Partnership working: building blocks

Partnerships as relationships

Strong personal relationships are based upon a partnership, as in a marriage, cohabitation or a civil partnership, and, to continue the analogy, one that is not forced and which has a clear purpose and remit. So it is with partnership working. A partnership in which the participants have no real idea why they are together, and no real motivation to continue and make a success of it, will be doomed. In a successful partnership, partners take 'partnership vows' after a courtship sequence and a rite of passage from being on their own to being together. In reality of course, just as in private relationships, partnerships cannot guarantee or sustain a lasting commitment: events often intervene.

Respecting respective contributions is another key factor in successful partnership working. One half of a couple might say, 'he makes our friends and I keep them': or a boss might credit his adviser – 'he does my thinking for me, and I present it'; or if you are a manager who cannot attend a key partnership meeting, a colleague from one of your partner agencies might say, 'I'll represent your interests for you if you can't be there', and you trust her to do so. Reciprocity can galvanise partnership working.

Interdependence

Partnership working always involves a degree of *interdependence*. Interdependence, or inter-relatedness, is when two or more people, or organisations, need each other and cannot function as well separately. Peter Gabbitas, Director of Health and Social Care Services for Edinburgh (a combined post with NHS Lothian) described how 'my "eureka moment" was when I realised early in my career that hospitals could not control the flow of acute admissions without working with other agencies' (quoted in *The Guardian* 2006).

Agencies may need one another in order to meet their own separate targets with government. Luton Council was able to recruit Asian administrators for the Bedfordshire police force as it had stronger links than the police into its local Asian communities (Douglas 2002). Given how much the police and many other public bodies struggle to make themselves feel attractive and safe as an employer to people from black and ethnic minority communities, recruitment is a key area for partnership working (Home Office data).

Even within competitive commercial contracts, interdependence plays its part. Postal distribution services within the UK are the subject of intense competition, yet by agreement between companies operating in the market, Royal Mail takes all post on the 'final delivery mile' to front doors. The public would not want two 'posties' from different companies coming up the front path or steps together, and it would be economically uncompetitive to do so, so companies collaborate. In a similar way, most goods and services are produced by a complex network of suppliers working together.

Interdependence is established when the sum of the whole in a partnership adds up to more than the sum of the parts, and partners realise that if they pull out, some crucial aspect of their performance will deteriorate as a direct result. As Hudson and Hardy say, 'a pre-requisite of partnership working is that potential partners have an appreciation of their interdependencies: without this appreciation, collaborative problem-solving makes no sense' (Hudson and Hardy 2002). This can include a failure to realize the impact of one organisation's actions upon another.

Few, if any, organisations are excellent in everything they do. Each has a gap in expertise or capacity, small or large, which another can help to fill. Models such as transaction cost theory can help to identify imperatives or incentives to collaborate (Hennart 2008).

Partnerships in the management of risks and resources

Managing risks to vulnerable individuals, along with managing limited resources, are the two major preoccupations for social care professionals today, irrespective of their sector or their employing organisation. Managing risk means living with the anxiety and actively managing a risk that someone vulnerable in contact with services may harm themselves, harm someone else, or be harmed by someone they know well. Managing resources is a constant anxiety in every social care agency. Despite record investment in social care in recent years, the gap between the available resources and those required remains considerable. Both of these factors – anxiety about risk and a shortage of resources – are reasons to develop partnership working and also reasons for its potential ineffectiveness.

The gathering momentum for partnership working

To coin a phrase, 'everyone's at it'. The range of practical applications of the partnership 'model' is huge:

* Nearly 40 per cent of architectural practices and 60 per cent of GP practices in the UK are partnerships.
* In 2003, Spain and Portugal entered a partnership to create a single Iberian electricity provider.
* Car sharing in cities is a fast-growing form of commuting.

Common social care risks, and the partnership actions that can reduce, though never completely eliminate, those risks

Three common risks

1   Serious violence to an individual inflicted by someone close to them
    Mitigation through partnership working
    • An accurate risk assessment, regularly updated (using central government, Local Safeguarding Children Board, Adult Protection Committee and individual agency guidelines).
    • A safety plan, setting out actions for family members and professionals (may include a professional visiting programme, behavioural or other treatment programmes, support groups).
    • Contingency arrangements in the event of rapid deterioration or crisis (emergency phone numbers, etc.).
    • A 'core group' of professionals *working together*, with a clearly assigned lead professional.

2   An irretrievable breakdown in personal functioning, with the potential to turn into a lasting mental health problem
    Mitigation through partnership working
    • Local capacity for immediate intervention by a psychiatrist, community psychiatric nurse (CPN) and an approved social worker (ASW), who are able to carry out a risk assessment, liaising with other professionals like the general practitioner, and who are able to organise any emergency medical treatment and/or social care package needed. NB: a mental health crisis can become acute within hours so a capacity for rapid response can limit damage.
    • Local availability of specialist resources e.g., for drug or alcohol related mental illness, for counselling.
    • Good joint working with children's services if a vulnerable adult is also a parent.

3   A frail older person discharged from hospital to go back home alone
    Mitigation through partnership working
    • A discharge plan agreed between the service user, professionals, family members and the members of a community support network, if there is one.
    • Provision of any equipment needed for safe community living e.g. walking aids, installations like rails or a stair lift to aid mobility within the home.
    • A community care package, perhaps home care, a meals service, a nursing service in the morning and at night, which goes in immediately the patient returns home.
    • Continuity of care between hospital and home.

- Three multi-national pharmaceutical companies have broken new ground by collaborating to produce the new 3-in-1 drug for HIV, Atripla.
- New superhighways are being built to link China, India, and Vietnam, collaborations between nations which would have been unthinkable 20 years ago.

All countries within the European Union have similar experiences and examples of partnership working across their social care services. They often share the process of getting there, too, even if some of their individual systems differ in emphasis or in how they are funded (Halloran 2000).

Everyday partnership working makes the world go round. Just to get to work in an average-sized town every day, thousands of citizens use the same pavements, roads, buses and trains in an orderly fashion, co-operating with each other, going about their business for the most part within a set of commonly understood and appreciated rules. Before going to work, in the privacy of peoples' homes, one person will use the bathroom first, someone will make the coffee, and perhaps someone else will lock the door behind them if they are the last to leave. In one of his novels, Ian McEwan writes:

> Henry thinks the city is a success, a brilliant invention, a biological masterpiece – millions teeming around the accumulated and layered achievements of the centuries, as though around a coral reef, sleeping working, entertaining themselves, harmonious for the most part, nearly everyone wanting it to work.
>
> (McEwan 2005)

You could write a book about partnership working simply by going anywhere in the world and observing street life for 24 hours. Amazing partnerships are being nurtured all the time between groups of friends, colleagues and loose acquaintances, united by a common cause or purpose. It is the same for social

---

Partnerships by the sea

Sixty fishermen working in two parallel lines of thirty spend two hours hauling a mile of rope in from the deep sea to retrieve their nets and the fish inside. As they tug on the rope, fighting with the undertow, they sing and chant to keep their morale high. The work is relentless but they always see through their shared task – all pulling in the same direction.

The learning point for social care teams is that often the task facing them needs to be simplified so everyone knows how to play their particular part in being successful – by all pulling in the same direction.

care professionals, where the ability to make instantly co-operative working relationships is crucial to getting it right on cases.

The human mind and body is the most awesome internal partnership of all.

> It starts with a single cell. The first cell splits to become two, the two become four and so on. After just 47 doublings, you have ten thousand trillion (10,000,000,000,000,000) cells in your body and are ready to spring forth as a human being. And every one of those cells knows exactly what to do to preserve and nurture you from the moment of your conception to your last breath.
>
> (Bryson 2003)

Many animal species demonstrate highly organised group behaviour, regulated by a phenomenal level of discipline within the group. Such behaviour is all the more important in hostile environments. Penguins in the Antarctic work in partnership to overcome great hardship and threats, memorably filmed by Luc Jacquet in *March of the Penguins* (Jacquet 2005). Jacquet's film illustrates the 'wisdom of crowds' and is one of the best films ever made about the principles of working together.

Social care partnerships also have to be synchronised, if not quite on that scale. One frail older woman, who is now in her nineties, has her own personalised care partnership: her informal carer next door who cooks for her, gets her up and puts her to bed; one of her daughters who lives in a nearby village and calls in most days to make sure she's OK; and other relatives who ring to keep in touch and reduce the social isolation that can accompany frailty like an invisible exclusion zone. The older woman is my mother-in-law.

Social care has been a hugely successful public service. 400,000 people now receive a state home care service, 280,000 a residential care service, and 30,000 people with disabilities now administer their own care using state money via a direct payment scheme – living proof of the large-scale and positive impact of a progressive movement and profession.

Partnership working: the enemies within

Partnership working is fashionable for good reasons, despite much spray-on rhetoric and the current tendency to chant 'partnership working' like a mantra, and to proclaim it as 'the new public sector cure-all' whenever something impossible needs doing quickly (CIPFA 2001). Saying partnership working is not the same as doing partnership working. Inflated claims and puffed-up posturing aside, partnership working is undoubtedly the only show in town when it comes to making a difference to complex social care problems.

However, the risks and downside of partnership working are just as powerful, including 'partnership overload' and 'partnership fatigue'. The potential for 'overdoing it' is a feature of business today, in either the public or private sector. For instance, a major UK electronics manufacturer is involved in 400 strategic alliances (Bamford *et al.* 2003), far too many to manage coherently.

Within the public sector, a plethora of new announcements and new initiatives combined with ongoing resource constraints are forcing many agencies to reduce all commitments they feel are at the margins of their work. For some, this means partnerships fall by the wayside.

And while stability is the holy grail of partnership leaders, relatively few partnerships can claim a secure enough infrastructure of personnel and systems to be guaranteed a long-term future in which they can settle down to concentrate on improving the quality of their services. Too many partnerships depend on a small number of key individuals – when they go, so does the partnership.

Partnership working also suffers from a lack of clarity and consistency in the use of eligibility criteria. The much bemoaned 'postcode lottery' for access to public services, is compounded by huge variability around the UK of who is referred to services and what action is then taken. For example, Baginsky found a wide variation between and within schools in respect of their willingness to report concerns about children to local authorities (Baginsky 2007).

Variations in eligibility also extend to inconsistency between age bands. A young person receiving a care package can have the level drastically cut when his or her case is transferred to an adult care services team. A 64-year-old in a small care home can sometimes be forced to transfer into sheltered housing from 65 onwards, because of different eligibility criteria and unequal levels of provision between age groups. I was once stranded in a lawless, ambiguous seven-mile no man's land between the Libyan and Algerian borders, wondering whose land I was actually in. It is like that for many people who use services. Stronger partnerships are needed across service boundaries if they are to avoid being experienced by people who use services as an unbridgeable gulf or chasm.

One thousand years into social care provision, it is a scandal that, despite the great efforts of over a million front-line social care staff, every minute of every day of every year, vulnerable people who use services are still forced to jump through hoops and hurdles or negotiate their way through confusing public sector mazes, just to get a basic service. Put simply, the service user experience is not good enough, or the 'failure to make progress locally is inexcusable: why should, say, organisational inertia, lack of leadership or professional protectionism be allowed to stand in the way of efficiency and quality gains that can be experienced directly by users? (Integrated Care Network 2008).

The point of partnership working is to end that.

References

Baginsky, M., 2007, 'Schools, social services and safeguarding children: past practice and future challenges', London: NSPCC (available at www.tinyurl.com/2cnagk).

Balloch, S. and Taylor, M., 2001, 'Can partnerships work?', in *Partnership Working: Policy and Practice*, Oxford: Policy Press.

Bamford J., Gomes Casseres, B. and Robinson, M., 2003, *Mastering Alliance Strategy*, San Francisco, CA: Jossey-Bass.

Bateman, N., 2006, *Practising Welfare Rights*, Oxon: Routledge.

Beresford P., 2005, 'What service users want', *The Guardian*, 23 March 2005.

Brown, Norman O., 1990, *Love's Body*, Berkeley, CA: University of California Press.

Bryson, B., 2003, *A Short History of Nearly Everything*, New York: Doubleday.

Cameron, A. and Masterson, A., 1998, 'The changing policy context of occupational therapy', *British Journal of Occupational Therapy*, 61(12): 556–60.

CIPFA, 2001, *Sterling Work: Financial Control and Budgeting for Local Authority Partnerships, A Practical Guide*, London: CIPFA.

Crawford, A., 1997, *The Local Governance of Crime: Appeals to Community and Partnerships*, Oxford: Oxford University Press.

CWDC, 2006, *Your Induction to Work in Children's Social Care: A Workbook for Those Working with Children, Young People and Their Families*, Leeds: CWDC.

DH, Home Office and DfEE, 1999, *Working Together to Safeguard Children: A Guide to Inter-Agency Working to Safeguard and Protect the Welfare of Children*, London: Department of Health, the Home Office and the Department of Education and Employment.

Douglas, A., June 2002, 'Is anybody out there: a study of recruitment and retention in social care in London', supplimentary report for the *Care in the Capital Campaign*.

Dowling, B., Powell, M. and Glendinning, C., 2004, 'Conceptualising successful partnerships', *Health and Social Care in the Community* 12: 309–17.

FAO, 2006, *Strengthening Co-Operatives for Sustainable Fisheries Management*, Costa Rica: Food and Agriculture Organisation.

Genn, H., Partington, M. and Wheeler, S., 2006, *Law in the Real World: Improving Our Understanding of How Law Works*, London: Nuffield Foundation.

Ghosh H., 2007, quoted in 'The green machine', *Whitehall and Westminster World*, May.

Gill, O. and Jack, G., 2000, 'Poverty and the child's world: assessing children's needs', *Poverty*, Winter 2000, London: Child Poverty Action Group.

Halloran, J. (ed.), 2000, *Building Partnerships for an Inclusive Europe*, Brighton: European Social Network.

Hennart, J.F., 2008, 'Transaction costs perspectives on inter-organisational relations', in S. Cropper, M. Ebers, C. Huxham and P. Smith Ring (eds) *The Oxford Handbook of Inter-Organisational Relations*, Oxford: Oxford University Press.

Hudson, B. and Hardy, B., 2002, 'What is a successful partnership and how can it be measured?' in C. Glendinning, M. Powell and K. Rummery (eds) *Partnerships, New Labour and the Governance of Welfare*, Oxford: Policy Press.

Huxham, C. and Vangen, S., 2005, *Managing to Collaborate: The Theory and Practice of Collaborative Advantage*, Oxon: Routledge.

Integrated Care Network, 2008, *Bringing the NHS and Local Government Together: A Practical Guide to Integrated Working*, London: Integrated Care Network (as part of the Care Services Improvement Partnership, Department of Health).

Jacquet L., 2005, *March of the Penguins* (DVD), Warner Films.

Kirk, S. and Glendinning, C., 2002, 'Supporting parents with a technology-dependent child', *Child Care, Health and Development*, 27(4): 321–34.

London Borough of Haringey, 2005, *Changing Lives: Tthe Children and Young People's Plan*, London: London Borough of Haringey.

McEwan, I., 2005, *Saturday*, London: Jonathan Cape, London.

Mill, J. and Church, D., 2006, *Safe learning*, London: Save the Children.

National Treatment Agency for Substance Misuse, 2005, *Developing Drug Services Policies*, No. 8, London: National Treatment Agency for Substance MisuseNational Treatment Agency 2002.

Powell, M. and Dowling, B., 2006, 'New Labour's partnerships: comparing conceptual models with existing forms', *Social Policy and Society*, 5(2): 305–14.

Sutton, K., 2005, 'Fighting fear of crime', *New Statesman*, 1 August.

Townsley, R., Watson, D. and Abbot, D., 2004, 'Working partnerships: A critique of the process of multi-agency working in services to disabled children with complex health care needs', *Journal of Integrated Care*, 12(2): 24–34.

2 The changing context for partnership working

> **Key messages**
> - Partnership working has a long history in the UK, and can lay claim to notable achievements
> - The forms it takes are now very different in England, Scotland, Wales and Northern Ireland
> - Service provision and service development lag behind fast-moving social, economic and technological trends, and the expectations of people who use services
> - Many partnerships are 'high maintenance': more than can be managed and supported properly

A short history of partnership working

From the very beginning

It is impossible to be precise about when partnership working in social care started. It has always been with us and always will be, which is both a truism and a recognition of its universality. Few early partnerships in social care are recorded, but that reflects the way social history has been written about as much as their absence. History has traditionally been studied through events, and there are few column inches in successful partnerships, even today. Collaboration between individuals or organisations to ease the plight of poor and vulnerable people was as concealed historically as it is now. As far as we know, the earliest communities took direct responsibility for those in their midst needing care, in some ways a state of affairs we are constantly striving to recapture.

The partly moral and partly tactical need for the government of the day in these islands to take some responsibility for the welfare and well-being of its people has been accepted for over a thousand years. Provision for the poor was made in common law for the first time during the reign of Athelstan, the first king of the English, who died in 940 AD. This reluctant partnership, in which the more able members of society part-funded the weakest through taxation, was based upon a mixture of genuine charity and the need to avoid social unrest. This continues to be the basis of social care today. The responsibilities of the state towards its citizens gathered pace in the Middle Ages, exercised through an increasingly well-connected network of churches and guilds. This culminated in a gradual and inexorable extension of the legal rights of citizens, interspersed with interludes of intense repression along the way, especially of minority groups. Dissent, also for the most part unrecorded, was always ruthlessly suppressed. Whilst an ad hoc responsibility was accepted for some vulnerable people, their treatment was often inhumane, as when people with severe mental health problems were put to sea for years in 'Ships of Fools'.

The first recorded social care partnerships were pioneering, such as the one between the painter William Hogarth, the composer George Friedrich Handel and the sea captain Thomas Coram, in the early eighteenth century. As he walked into London from his home in Rotherhithe, Coram was distressed and horrified to see the corpses of abandoned babies by the roadside. Hogarth helped Coram to fund the Foundling Hospital in Holborn, which opened in 1741 as the first residential school for children. Coram children were the first in the world to be systematically inoculated and the first to be taken on holiday every year. Hogarth painted Coram and Handel wrote a 'Performance of Vocal and Instrumental Musick' to raise money (Pugh 2007). Handel's Foundling Anthem, 'blessed are they that considereth the poor', was aimed at potential donors. All this stood in stark contrast to the punitive culture of the workhouses, in which:

> a great many poor Infants, and exposed Bastard Children, are inhumanly suffered to die by the Barbarity of Nurses, especially Parish Nurses, who are a sort of People void of Commiseration, or Religion; hired by the Churchwardens to take off a Burthen from the Parish at the cheapest and easiest Rates they can; and these know the Manner of doing it effectually, as by the Burial Books may evidently appear.
>
> (Journals of the House of Commons, 1 March 1715)

This early form of commissioning by parishes show how sometimes, without a strong value base and effective regulation, public-sector commissioners can be tempted to choose the cheapest possible way of pushing a problem out of sight.

By the start of the nineteenth century, following the American and French revolutions, the pressure for social change could no longer be contained. The British establishment either had to make substantial reforms or itself be faced with revolution. There were other factors. The absence of strategy and regulation was leading to an uncontrolled expansion of slums in towns like Nottingham – towns which were growing fast and attracting economic migrants, as many UK cities still do today. Leaving the administration of the Poor Law at the local level meant that parish rates increased dramatically towards the end of the eighteenth century in many parts of the country, to the disgust of most parishioners. The system also offered little if any protection to the vulnerable. Of 2,339 children received into the London workhouses between 1750 and 1755, only 168 were alive in 1755. Although charities filled some of the gaps, providing good care for the few while the state provided poorer care for the many, the need for government to develop social care policy was becoming compelling.

Throughout the nineteenth and early twentieth centuries, charities in the form of voluntary organisations began to evolve a more organised model of social care. This eventually led to the co-operative movement, with new partnerships like credit unions advocating and often pump-priming financial inclusion. The co-operative model has contemporary applications, such as the wider remit taken on by the Leeds City Credit Union (see box below), and the first nationwide communities of interest credit unions, being developed by the Family Fund for families of children with disabilities, in partnership with True Colours and the Esmeé Fairbairn Foundation. Member-led movements have a long tradition in the UK, starting with the Rochdale pioneers, 28 local people who opened the first co-operative shop in 1844. The co-operative movement today is based in over 100 countries with over 800 million members. Member-led movements are social partnerships which as well as providing services, aim to further the interests of their members. Hence the early co-operative movement focused particularly on education, as the means of supporting their members' aspirations for upward social mobility.

Leeds City Credit Union

Credit unions are financial co-operatives, owned and controlled by their members, originally formed in order to make low-cost loans available to local people who were short of funds, unable to qualify for bank loans and who were often at the mercy of loan sharks. Credit unions are supported by the Association of British Credit Unions Ltd (ABCUL) and the Financial Services Authority (FSA), and are an example of local partnership working in practice.

In 2001, the Leeds City Credit Union expanded its membership from current or former employees of the City Council, to include everyone living in Leeds, which makes it the largest credit union approved by the FSA. Its services include banking, low-cost insurance, the full range of financial services, and affordable credit for its members. It has a Young Savers scheme for under-16s and is a good example of a membership organisation founded on principles of mutualism and keeping this principle intact through successive periods of social change.

Employee share-ownership schemes and co-owned firms are clear modern alternatives to traditional corporate structures. The Mondragon network in the Basque region of Spain is the most successful co-operative structure in the developed world, with over 160 co-operatives, 30,000 worker-members, and annual sales of £5 billion dollars. Grameen Bank is 90 per cent controlled by 7.4 million clients. In the United States, employee stock ownership (ESOP) makes a 'substantial contribution to community stabilisation', with total worker holdings amounting to 8 per cent of all US corporate stock by the late 1990s, for a total of £800 billion dollars (Williamson *et al.* 2003).

Partnership working since the 1970s

Partnership working entered the social care *Zeitgeist* in the 1970s, for four main reasons. The first was the result of advocacy by many leading professionals in the 1950s and 1960s, who foresaw the need for more joint working – new developments are invariably preceded by a period of intense campaigning, whose significance can be subsequently overlooked.

The second was a realisation that the big social care issues of the day needed much more than changes in legislation and new investment. Legitimate and overdue expectations for de-institutionalisation – a professional *cri de coeur* for the thousands of people of all ages unfairly and unnecessarily detained in residential children's homes, long-stay hospitals and care homes to be returned to the community, ironically often to the very community that rejected them in the first place – could only be met through concerted inter-agency action over two to three decades.

The third reason was the lower growth rate of the UK economy in the 1970s and 1980s which made it harder to sustain ever-increasing levels of public expenditure. The call for the public sector to restrain spending and spend what there was in a wiser way became louder.

The fourth reason was a step change in awareness, fuelled by research and practice experience, of the dangers vulnerable people who use services were being exposed to in their own homes and sometimes in state care. Accompanying this was a related appreciation of the systemic complexity of many situations the state knew it should be intervening in, and the realisation there were too few staff, too little training and too few resources available to make a lasting difference unless working practices changed dramatically.

The development of partnerships to tackle organised child abuse

Over the past 30 years, the methods of tackling organised child abuse have changed beyond recognition. In the 1960s and 1970s, the Paedophile Information Exchange was an organisation through which paedophiles communicated with each other in a relatively open way. It hitched itself to the counter-cultural movement of the late 1960s, hiding the serious and systematic abuse of children under a cloak of libertarian rhetoric. When child abuse was suspected within families, concerned parents and relatives took what informal steps they could to keep their children safe, such as absenting themselves from family gatherings. Little was known about sexual abuse and its impact upon children until individual social workers and groups within the women's movement began to draw attention to the dangers of paedophile activity and organised abuse within networks of abusing adults. Information about what happened in those dark decades for children is still coming to light for the first time today. The safeguarding authorities, themselves struggling to build up a knowledge base, sometimes belittled concerns and sometimes over-reacted, as in Cleveland and the Orkneys, where, respectively, sexual abuse and ritual abuse were wrongly thought to be present at epidemic levels. As a result, large groups of children were wrongly taken into care as suspected abuse victims. Yet despite occasional excesses, numerous inquiries subsequently have shown how right professionals were to be concerned. This has helped to stop the pendulum drifting back again into a new era of non-intervention, as well as acting as a constraint on over-zealous professionals.

In the 1990s, a number of paedophiles were finally brought to justice, although some criminal cases collapsed due to a lack of conclusive evidence. The importance of facilitating children to give evidence in court, including via video link, was gradually understood and more child-centred procedures were developed. New multi-agency public protection panels (MAPPAs) were put in place to monitor paedophiles who presented a continuous danger to children and young people.

The murders in 2002 of the 10-year-old schoolgirls Holly Wells and Jessica Chapman in Soham, Cambridgeshire by their school caretaker Ian Huntley, led, following the Bichard Inquiry, to tighter national systems for transferring intelligence about suspected paedophiles between police forces and local authorities, though implementation of this initiative, deemed essential and urgent at the time, became patchier with the passage of time.

In 2006, the first successful prosecution against a UK paedophile for abusing children in another country, Ghana, was brought against Alexander Kilpatrick under the 2003 Sexual Offences Act. A major global police operation, Operation Ore, led to the conviction of many adults who had systematically downloaded child pornography onto their computers in different countries.

In 30 years, knowledge about how paedophiles operate, and how to stop them, had been transformed through a succession of partnerships involving assessment and enforcement agencies. This was achieved despite the intrinsic continuing difficulties in monitoring the way people move around the country and world at will, and the innate difficulty of stopping abuse within families, where control is often maintained by the abuser/s in a tyrannical and violent way, and where investigators typically encounter deception and subterfuge.

The need for further change

Changing the working culture

Although the importance of partnership working was becoming appreciated and accepted, the frameworks for putting it into practice were either cumbersome or non-existent. A strong sense of status and hierarchy meant that networking up and down the lines of management and across organisations was often seen by senior managers in organisations as wrongly bypassing superiors or 'sleeping with the enemy'. The tendency for decisions to be delegated upwardly led to wholesale disempowerment on the front line, with staff often having to make lengthy bureaucratic submissions to gain approval for minor decisions. Stodgy joint committees – for instance the Joint Consultative Committees (JCCs), which sat between the local NHS and council(s) – met every few months during the 1970s and most of the 1980s, but rarely took major decisions even in respect of obviously overlapping public health issues. Emergency duty services, training consortia and Area Child Protection Committees, were early forerunners of partnership working, but they were fringe activities.

Writing in 2004 about joint working across the Irish border regions, Donaghy and McReynolds concluded that 'in assessing progress to date, it is important to recall that only 15 years ago, cross-border co-operation in health and community care on the island of Ireland was almost non-existent, apart from isolated ventures involving small numbers of patients' (Donaghy and McReynolds 2004). This comment could equally well apply to most areas of the mainland UK. 'Lift off' for partnership working has only really taken place in the last fifteen years. During that period, growth has been exponential, although to some extent, what ever fixed point you take in time, developments appear radical compared to what went before.

Change in the status quo was desperately needed. For example, services rarely met the needs of black and minority ethnic communities, despite people who use services from those communities being disproportionately represented, especially in services like mental health. Nor did they meet the needs of a growing number of people with disabilities for decent support in the community like adapted social housing. It became clear to many academics, practitioners and civil servants working in the field that making partnership working a formal requirement would offer the best route to deliver social policies with a limited political and public popularity.

Regime change in the late 1980s and 1990s

Since the late 1980s, stronger national arrangements for partnership working have been established, such as youth offending teams (YOTs) operating under the auspices of the Youth Justice Board, as set out in the 1998 Crime and Disorder Act. Youth offending was previously dealt with as part of the main care system for children and young people, which meant too few specialist services were developed. Set up as joint teams, with social workers, police officers, probation offices and education welfare officers as core team members, YOTs helped to break down inter-professional divisions, although they risked becoming a new silo themselves.

In the 1990s, the greater focus on spending money wisely and producing continuous efficiency savings grew into a preoccupation, with a number of seminal Audit Commission studies and inspection reports showing that public services were often inefficient, ineffective, and not *value for money*. A regime change started to emerge that was based on a less politicised managerial culture, accompanied by a curtailment of trade union influence and a shift to a service-user first rather than a staff-first belief system – sometimes described as 'New Public Management'. However, this paradigm shift brought with it some significant downsides, such as the virtual collapse of a model of relationship-based social work.

The limitations of regime change

Despite great efforts to reduce it by a succession of different political administrations, public expenditure continued to grow throughout the 1990s, and from 1997 a more expansionist Labour government took spending to higher levels than ever before. However, this still did not bring complete relief. The inescapable reality is that care for those most in need is very expensive. For example, the cost in 2007 to Westminster Council of looking after ten children with particularly complex needs was £3 million, the equivalent of supporting hundreds of families through family support programmes. The difficulty has always been that those ten children have to be looked after as the first priority of Westminster and other local authorities facing the same dilemma is to comply with its statutory responsibility. Increasingly, costly packages of care are being distilled to an ever-diminishing group of people, despite government policy to make services universally available and accessible. The difficulty switching resources from acute or heavy-end services to preventative services is the same in the health service, where acute care continues to dominate overall expenditure compared to community health services (Ham 2004).

Political impetus towards partnership working

Two political developments were instrumental in the growth of partnership working. The first, during the third and fourth terms of the 1979–1997 Conservative government, was to introduce a market mentality into social care. This chased the coat tails of the 'purchaser/provider' split in the NHS, introducing compulsory competitive tendering (CCT) for many public services, and the notion of *best value*. Whilst much of social care provision was initially exempted from this regime, some social care authorities redefined themselves as strategic commissioning authorities, outsourcing most of their directly provided services, either to the private sector or to arms-length management companies, as in Cumbria and Hertfordshire. They were ten to fifteen years ahead of their time, as every social care authority now defines itself in terms of its strategic commissioning role.

The growing service user movement and pressure groups helped to accelerate the adoption of a commissioning function, albeit from left field as many commentators questioned the relevance of the pure market model to the NHS and to social care services. As Bill Jordan said 'services are not commodities: they involve "relational goods" of affection, respect and belonging – we are not running a supermarket' (Jordan 2006). In fact, first into the supermarket were people who use services. Social care professionals found that they had under-estimated their level of discontent with mainstream service provision.

The second significant political development was the incoming Labour government's determination from 1997 onwards to deal more effectively with chronic social problems such as child poverty and social exclusion. Frank Dobson, the new Secretary of State for Health spoke and wrote forcefully about bringing down what he disparagingly referred to as the 'Berlin Wall' between health and social services. In 2000, the NHS Plan contained a whole chapter about partnership working and development – unprecedented in a public strategy document.

This tougher approach brought with it a much stronger performance assessment regime run through national inspectorates, including a formidable target culture. Some organisations went from having no targets at all to hundreds, within five years. Some of these targets were always going to be impossible to achieve, such as reducing serious drug use by 50 per cent between 1998 and 2003. However, the political ambition concentrated professional minds on both the quantity and quality of the services they were commissioning and providing, whereas these had too often been taken for granted. This is the political and policy context for today's much more intensive partnership working.

Partnerships today

Partnerships galore

The last ten years have witnessed a bewildering array of new partnerships, some disappearing from sight almost as soon as they were established. Health Improvement Programmes; Education Action Zones; Health Action Zones; Early Years Development and Childcare Partnerships; GP fundholding, all were introduced, then rapidly superseded. Many partnership vehicles ahead of their time in the 1990s, like the Independent Living Fund, now find themselves behind the times, with the development of individual budgeting for people with disabilities. The pace of change at a policy level can be contrasted with the snail-like pace of change on the ground for many people who use and depend on services.

Many new organisations were not given long enough to succeed, the most extreme example being the National Care Standards Commission (NCSC),

---

Learning disability services: a positive and lasting transformation

The transformation of learning disability services has been a major strategic achievement of the last 25 years.

Until the 1970s/80s, learning disability services had little status in either the NHS or local authorities, despite many people having the potential to lead ordinary lives if well supported. Many were placed in long-stay hospitals or unregistered residential care homes, in which neglect, and sometimes an abusive culture, went unchecked. People with similar or even greater disabilities lived at home, supported by members of their family who received little recognition of their own needs as 24/7 carers. In the 1990s, programmes like 'Valuing People', and 'Supporting People' injected more funding, status and inter-agency working into learning disability services. The NHS made capital funding available in order to close many long-stay hospitals and reprovide them with supported housing units, usually on the same sites to make planning permission easier to secure, although in the process reinforcing the isolation of the residents from their local community. Over the same period, joint community learning disability teams were established, with NHS clinical staff such as specialist nurses and psychologists coming alongside local authority social workers and care managers as core team members. Each area had a Learning Disability Partnership Board in place, often co-chaired by a senior manager and a person using services role-modelling 'working together'. By 2003, Partnership Board meetings were open to the press and public in Manchester, Surrey, Northamptonshire, Nottingham, Warwickshire and St Helens (Mencap 2003).

Local government took the lead role with learning disability, as did the NHS for mental health services, where similar programmes were established. By 2009, local authorities will have complete responsibility for learning disability services, completing the sea-change from a medical to a social model of learning disability. This shift means that actions plans for specific issues facing people with learning disabilities can be more easily developed. One example is concerted action to screen for and tackle obesity, levels of which are higher than for the general population, at 35 per cent compared with 22 per cent (Kerr 2004).

which only lasted 17 days before its successor body, the Commission for Social Care Inspection (CSCI) was announced. Such Darwinian politics led to the survival of the fittest, or sometimes the survival of the most politically astute. Endless competitive repositioning took place, especially by boards and senior management teams. A by-product was that some professional groups continued to work within out-of-date frameworks, because they did not realise a further change had taken place. They decided the best strategy was to bury their head in the sand, ignore all the changes, and try as best as they could to get on with the day job. If this sounds half-empty, a half-full version is that change was sorely needed, and that each new programme incorporated and built on the part-proven benefits of previous programmes.

The momentum for service development had been successfully driven forward by a disparate yet ideologically united critical mass of professional staff and service-user champions and representatives. However, it is worth noting that achievements often carry their own limitations: the new community services for people with learning disabilities, much favoured by older people who use services, who never thought they would experience them in their lifetime, have since been rejected by many younger learning disabled people. They see these community services as being too based around day centres and other group care models, which are out of step with the more flexible and personalised ways in which they wish to live their lives. What was normal – even aspirational – for one generation had become abnormal and unacceptable for the next.

Similar transformations took place in services like drug and alcohol services, and youth justice services, now organised through local multi-agency Drug Action Teams and Youth Offending Teams respectively. However, there is no guarantee that investment in a service will be maintained at the same level, especially if an issue plummets down the political agenda. Campaigners and people who use services claim that HIV services, which were well funded in the early 1990s, are now in a state of neglect (Weatherburn *et al.* 2007).

Partnership working: the legal position

The statutory definition of partnership describes it rather archaically, mostly for company law and tax purposes, as 'the relation which subsists between persons carrying on a business with a view of profit.' Partnerships are governed by the Partnership Act 1890 (Martin and Law 2006). The only update to this simple overarching legal framework in the last ten years has been the Limited Liability Partnership Act 2000, which sought to give more flexibility to partners, especially in businesses consisting of mixed professions or disciplines, to give confidence about managing the start-up risks involved. Regulations are as important as legislation, particularly those procurement regulations which reflect European Union directives and require a good contract lawyer to interpret. Government guidance in the form of policies and procedures like National Service Frameworks also convey advice in the form of high-level guidance for making professional judgements. However, the way in which more than 1.4 million staff in social care, one in 20 of the working population in the UK and 15 per cent of the public service workforce (CSCI *et al.* 2007), apply the range of advice, guidance and instructions about partnership working requirements remains individualised and idiosyncratic.

Section 75 of the NHS Act 2006 – formerly s31 of the Health Act 1999 – is the only act of parliament in England allowing statutory organisations to set up pooled budgets through so-called 'Health Act flexibilities'. Scotland has parallel provision in the Community Care and Health (Scotland) Act 2002. The risks of going beyond this, even in pursuit of a partnership working goal, can be potentially serious – the council-owned London Authorities Mutual Ltd (LAML) was challenged in the High Court by the insurance firm Risk Management Partners (RMP), who claimed the councils acted beyond their legal powers. On 22 April 2008, judgement was given in favour of LAML. Some London councils claimed they satisfied the 'Teckal exemption', which means they do not have to go through a full procurement process, and this point is yet to be ruled upon at the time of writing.

Notifications to the respective governments about new pooled budgeting arrangements were slow to begin with, as they are with any new provision, but accelerated after 2002. In fact by 2002, there were 63 pooled budgets in English mental health services with a combined value of £800 million, which was a rapid take-up in historical terms. Section 75 of the NHS Act 2006 also allows a secretary of state to order a 'directed partnership arrangement', where an inquiry or an inspection has shown the absence of partnership working to be a contributory cause of service failure. The Children Act 2004 encouraged the formation of Children's Trusts, under the local leadership of a Director of Children's Services, as did the Health and Social Care Act 2001 in respect of Care Trusts for adult services, both subject to Secretary of State approval. Through the 'Putting People First' programme for adult social care services, local authorities have to demonstrate progress on facilitating self-directed care, including personal budgets for people who use services. Progress will be measured by the regulator CSCI – which is being replaced from April 2009 by the Care Quality Commission (CQC) – through a new national performance indicator.

Legal constraints continue to curb the extent and potential of full partnership working. It is generally not possible for one agency to delegate its powers and functions to another. Most partnership boards and other joint governance structures have no executive authority or decision-making power – which increases the importance of partnership working and joint agreements. Those local authorities and health authorities who have wanted to form a Local Public Service Trust, thereby taking the widest possible approach to integrating local public services, could not do so without a further – and unlikely – change in primary legislation. In a parliamentary answer on 12 September 2007, the English Health Secretary, Alan Johnson, confirmed that English local authorities could not make and pay for residential care placements in Scotland and Northern Ireland, and under s21 of the National Assistance Act 1948, could only place people in England and Wales. The inability to make cross-border placements for people who live for example in the north of Northumberland, is a strong argument to update all current legislation to facilitate the maximum possible degree of partnership working.

The impact of devolution on partnership working models in the UK

In 1998, *Tackling Drugs Together* was published, aimed at reversing a worrying social trend and aiming ultimately to build a Britain free of hard drugs. If the same document were published in 2008 by the UK government, it could only be applied to England, not to the whole of the United Kingdom. The Welsh Assembly Government, the Scottish Government and the Northern Ireland Executive, now put their own national stamp on law, policies and services. For example, the development of the Legislative Competence Order for vulnerable children in Wales will allow Wales to develop its own primary legislation for the first time. Irreversible devolution has replaced an ambivalence towards decentralisation, and the earlier tension in the 1997 Blair government, between *dirigisme* and pluralism (Marquand 1998) has given way to a politically sensitive co-existence, complicated by multiple changes in governments across the UK.

Legislators in Wales and Scotland have preferred to develop stronger joint working arrangements, placing an emphasis on voluntary co-operation, rather than the English predilection for wholesale structural change. This has led to the promotion of stronger networks such as ' managed care networks' for older people (Hudson 2007). Having been asked by the Scottish Executive to review the future of the NHS in Scotland, Kerr described the English obsession with structures as 'like pre-Machiavellian Italy with warring Italian states ... it's warfare, not working together' (Kerr 2005). The Welsh Health Minister, Brian Gibbons, said:

> We think that our public services in Wales will be best delivered on the basis of partnership, co-operation and collaboration, not commercialisation, competition, outsourcing and privatisation. We need to get our public services working more closely together with a shared responsibility for delivering care to the individual and to the community. It is a distinctive model, based on Welsh values and needs, and the opportunity has been given to us by devolution to allow us to deliver it here in Wales.

> (Gibbons 2007)

Rhodes saw this as moving to 'self-organising inter-organisational networks' (Rhodes 1997).

The pace of change quickens yet again

This Cook's tour of the history of social care partnerships ends with the position in early 2008, which is as exciting, confusing and as volatile as ever. Additional duties of partnership on local government in England are being introduced in a new Local Government and Public Involvement in Health Act 2007. New joint duties in the Childcare Act (2006) have paved the way for stronger joint working between JobCentre Plus and Children's Centres to ensure an adequate supply of child care places. Within the health service, all NHS Provider Trusts must either become Foundation Trusts or Social Enterprise Companies by the end of 2008, the latest of a wave of reorganisations in the NHS which have left many participants disoriented. Within the justice system, a new joint duty between the civil service (through Her Majesty's Courts Service (HMCS) and the judiciary (through the Lord Chief Justice), aimed at making the courts in England and Wales work more efficiently, brings together agencies who have traditionally been constitutionally independent of each other into a more pragmatic proximity in order to solve a chronic set of problems. And lastly, a glut of major reviews have either reported recently or are due to in the near future, with all calling for better partnership working. These include: the Leitch Review of future working population skills; the Lyons Reviews of public sector financing and devolution of some public sector nerve centres from London; the Gershon review of efficiency savings; the Varney Review of public sector reform to make it more customer-centric; and the Wanless reviews of NHS and social care funding needs over the next generation.

The rhetoric about joint working goes on, still way ahead of the reality. In his introduction to the White Paper on the future of NHS Community Services, *Our Health, Our Care, Our Say*, published in January 2006, Prime Minister Tony Blair said 'These changes will be matched by much better links between health and social care' (Department of Health 2006). The echo of Frank Dobson's long-ago reference to 'a Berlin Wall coming down', is a reflection that the long haul in partnership working is about cultural change between and within organisations which can take decades, and which structural change can either help or hinder. The levers available to central Governments are limited, the more so as society becomes more complex and fragmented. Nye Bevan and Herbert Morrison, the key Labour ministers in the post-war Attlee government, constructed the modern NHS in a few months in 1946, to start in 1948. No politician or politicians could achieve such a level of change so quickly today (Beckett 1997).

The reason primary legislation is often a last resort when trying to develop partnerships is the amount of time and effort it takes to put a single Bill on the statute book, let alone implement it. A vast number of specialists, inside and outside government, work together to shape a single Bill and subsequently, an Act of Parliament. Academics, business representatives, professional associations, trade unions, parliamentarians and specialist civil servants, numbering on average between 50 and 100, will work together in different ways over a number of months to draft a single piece of new legislation.

Partnership working in a changing world

Responding to social change

Partnerships need to keep pace with the times and to reflect wider changes in society, particularly more complex patterns of inter-connectivity and inter-relatedness. To paraphrase John Donne, no public service is an island. Transition is the new natural state. More people are in transition – between relationships, jobs and countries. Transition communities are towns and villages with a commitment to long-term sustainable housing, water supply, low electricity use, and other resource-reducing programmes. Patterns of care are becoming briefer and more intensive. For example, care episodes are getting shorter. On average, an older person stays in an old people's home for fifteen months, compared to three times as long five years ago. This reflects a change in the threshold for entering residential care, with those entering today being far more frail than a generation ago. The average duration of time in care for a child is five years, with fewer children entering care but staying longer. To respond to these societal shifts, social care services have to become less linear, more flexible and more diverse. Services have to be ready to respond to needs that are increasingly diverse, at short notice and with a minimum of delay.

This is mirrored by shorter attention spans, resulting in the average length of a scene in a television soap being cut by over fifty per cent in the last few years, by the rise in interim management and, in social care, by workers choosing to stay on the books of agencies instead of permanent employers – trends which involve less attachment to a stable employer, more preparedness to take risks, and, disturbingly for those people who use services and who value practitioner continuity, employment options which guarantee a way out from a team or caseload that doesn't suit or which is going wrong. Rapid change is concisely expressed in a story told by the Secretary of State for Children Schools and Families, Ed Balls, about a child he had met who berated his grandmother for 'using twentieth century techniques on twenty-first century children'.

The speed of change means that young people view the world very differently from young adults only ten years older than them. In this sense, generation gaps are both multiplying and reducing, with greater gulfs between closer-spaced generations, not so much between young and old, but between 15-year-olds and 25-year-olds, and between 25 and 35-year-olds, and so on. This comes through when I have discussed concerns about identity and community with teenage gang members.

Time-scales in partnerships are complex. It is hard for partners' time-scales to match one another as, invariably, one has more pressing problems than the other(s). The timelines in private finance initiative (PFI) contracts are especially hard to mesh. Investors and providers need a regular and predictable repayment schedule, whereas commissioners often try to change or vary the specification of what is provided. The commissioning authority may experience a change in political control or management during the lifetime of the contract, leading to a fundamental change of policy or attitude towards the PFI partner. These 'trajectory changes' are one factor in the weakening of interest in long-term PFI deals, and an increase in wariness about the organisational and financial risks involved.

Partnership working also has to keep pace with change at the level of personal identity, in which individuals are bombarded with both attacks on their identity and opportunities to re-invent themselves. These trends can be understood through the concept of *intersectionality*, which focuses on multiple identities and the multiple social categories to which people now belong. Intersectionality is the science of the cross-over between various factors such as race, ethnicity, culture and religion as they apply to an individual.

Responding to demographic and technological change

Dramatic population trends are defining the need for future partnerships. Some cities in China, like Shenzhen (13.3 million), Tianjin (11.5 million) and Cheng Du (11 million), are virtually unheard of in the West, yet already have populations the size of London, 'filling the dreams of businessmen from Sydney to San Francisco – the 1 billion customers, the 1 billion new capitalists, the 1 billion market place' (Parsons 2008). In the UK, there will be 25 per cent more people over 65 by 2017, and 38 per cent more over 85, with consequential rises in age-related disability. The proportion of children in single-parent households tripled between 1972 and 2004 and now stands at 24 per cent. The fastest growing group of new householders are single women in their thirties, economically independent enough for the first time to make major life choices for themselves. The 310,000 marriages and 161,000 divorces a year in the UK have implications for the future of social housing and children in need services. There are four times as many widows as widowers, with unspecified service requirements. 'Demographics' presents both commissioners and providers of social care with great challenges. The oldest grandparent caring for a child and in touch with the Grandparents Association for support is 89, bringing up her great granddaughter, and the youngest is 28, bringing up her granddaughter. The average age of a grandparent in the UK today is younger than expected at 46 (The Grandparents Association).

Technological change is equally significant. Eighty per cent of households in the UK have access to a home computer and one-third of all school children have the internet in their bedroom, showing the need or simply the opportunity for more online social care services and, in the case of children, the need for online security – the Child Exploitation and Online Protection (CEOP) police service asks the open question 'who are the key partners in the online world?'. Online services cover every aspect of modern life. Registered users of specialist websites like www.singlemuslim.com and www.shaadi.com arrange their own traditional Muslim marriage. The number of subscribers doubled between 2006 and 2007. And for those who may scoff at the idea of social care services being provided online, be warned: 89 per cent of Kooth (www.kooth.com) users – an online counselling and support service for young people – say they prefer online counselling to telephone support, an unsurprising statistic for children reared on text messaging who often use thumbs instead of their index fingers to press doorbells, and who now often struggle with written exams and assessments because handwriting is an alien concept.

It would be difficult to discuss demographic change without noting the huge change in the ethnic mix in some areas within the UK. In some parts of the country, black and ethnic minority communities are now 'the majority community', even though they are not one community but several. In some inner London boroughs, over 200 languages are spoken within a few square miles.

Service providers have rarely developed their services quickly enough to meet community needs as they arise. Inevitably there are resource implications. Whilst council spending on care rose by 65 per cent between 1997 and 2006, government grants have only increased by 14 per cent, with the high level of council expenditure unsustainable in the longer-term given likely tighter budget settlements (LGA figures in *Without a care?* (2006) and statistics from the Office of National Statistics (ONS), the Government Actuary's Department, the General Register Office for Scotland and the Northern Ireland Statistics and Research Agency').

The partnership implications of these demographic changes are considerable, and need to be on the mainstream agenda for Children's Trusts and Health and Care Trusts. Mapping out the broad groups of services needed for 2020 or 2025, and planning coherently to bring them about, is essential. The massive workforce development and technological challenge involved will require the involvement of many specialist partners in carefully constructed contracts of up to ten to 20 years in length. The partnership between commissioning agencies and their local taxpayers will also need strengthening as taxes will almost certainly have to rise locally over the next two decades to meet an expanding and more diverse set of community needs and social pressures.

The personalisation agenda

At the level of individual access to social care services, a fundamental change has been taking place, known as 'personalisation', which has parallels with developments in other sectors such as health care with the growth of 'theranostics' – personalised medicine based on a test designed to predict whether a particular patient will benefit from a standard treatment. The self-advocacy organisation, In Control, sets out six governing principles for personalisation: self-determination, direction, money, home, support and community life, to underpin service strategies (Duffy 2008). These principles are matched by the seven Common Core Principles for social workers, to support self-care (Department of Health 2008).

As a consequence of rising incomes, which translates into more consumer purchasing power, many individuals have increased choice both about what to buy, and about their stake in public services. An increasing number of organisations are providing citizens with information which was previously the exclusive province of governments. Early in 2008, the BBC Radio 4 programme, 'You and Yours' developed an online 'care calculator' to show the average level of state-funded care available in different parts of the UK. This enabled anyone who might need to use services in different parts of the country to see how the level of provision in their local area compared with others. This added to the growing criticism of restrictive eligibility criteria. Concerns about people who fail to gain access to social care despite having significant support needs was a central theme of the annual report on the *State of Social Care* from the Commission for Social Care Inspection (CSCI 2008).

Personalisation has been identified as an explicit objective of government policy for adult social care. The publication in December 2007 of a concordat (*Putting People First*) announced a shared vision and commitment to the transformation of adult social care. A key aspect of this will be that person-centred planning and self-directed support become mainstream, with personal budgets on offer for everyone eligible for publicly funded adult social care support (HM Government 2007). This will increasingly involve working with people who use services and with their families and carers as key partners in the co-production of care and support. Lord Darzi's review of the NHS has also indicated that in future personal budgets – including NHS resources – might be available to people with long-term conditions. These changes could have profound impact on the nature of local authority social care and the role of social workers. Increasingly it is expected that there will be less social care time spent on assessment (not least because of the primacy of self-assessment), and more on support, brokerage and advocacy.

Personalisation for adults who need support has ramifications beyond the social care world. Increasingly the focus is on 'wellbeing' and addresses people's needs in a more rounded and holistic manner. This has been facilitated, for example in the Individual Budget (IB) pilots undertaken in 13 English councils (an independent evaluation report was due for publication in the summer of 2008) which have integrated funding streams from a range of sources in addition to social care. It is not only the funding which is different, but also the process and nature of the support that might be organised. With the guiding focus being on the *outcomes* that are to be achieved for an individual, the means of delivering this might include a range of universal and open access services, including leisure, education, housing, transport etc, as well as services that might be recognised as 'social care'.

Personalisation is as much a theme of current social care as it is of contemporary lifestyles, with blogs, video diaries and customised, tailored products, even funerals. In 2007, I went to the funeral of a colleague who had scripted the poems, prayers and songs for the service before she died. The ceremony was conducted by an independent celebrant, with the crematorium itself merely a borrowed space in which to conduct a personalised ceremony.

Another example of a personalised service is child-inclusive mediation after parental separation or divorce. In this model, children are included in discussions about what happens to them, rather than this being either fought out or mediated exclusively between the parents. 'I was able to say what I wanted without feeling sad or worrying about making other people feel sad', and 'It's made everything easier, mum and dad don't fight so much. Now I can say what I want to say without being told I am wrong' (children, 12 and 11 respectively, quoted in Goldson 2006).

However, as with most new policies, the rhetoric outstrips the reality. Reviews of personalisation programmes in social care point to the implementation challenges, particularly access and facilitation (Henwood and Hudson 2007).

New models of partnership in leadership and management are also appearing, such as co-headships, in which a principal of a school works alongside an executive head, who is responsible for overseeing a small group of schools. This can be particularly supportive to a new head, who can be mentored on the job by someone with more experience.

Choice is being increasingly extended across society – for instance in the way colleges of all descriptions now provide flexible personalised learning programmes and in the way a larger number of employers allow employees to work more flexibly, to support them as far as possible with a work–life balance, not least because promoting such flexibility is now a legal requirement, in legislation like the Work and Families Act 2006.

But while personalised support services are scaling up, the choices offered do not yet extend as far as offering a choice of practitioner, or a choice of placement. The NHS is moving in this direction with the publication of individual consultant success rates in the health service. That time may come in social care. Further change cannot come quickly enough for Alan, who told me, 'I have had to go back to the same place for respite care five years running, because that's where my local authority has a contract. Most people would not like to keep going back to the same place every year. I would like more choice too.'

Personalisation needs considerable resourcing. It takes much more time getting to know individuals than it does to pigeonhole them and to make assumptions about them as members of a particular social group, family religion or community. In thinking about working with individuals, specific practice models can help, such as One Plus One's focus on the 'turn to' moment, when a counsellor and a client reach a breakthrough in understanding, and a shift in thinking. This happened to me in my early twenties, still trying to make sense of an unhappy adoption, which I had been acting out in various ways. I started to read a book called *Ego, Hunger and Aggression*, by Fritz Perls, in Compendium Bookshop in Camden Town, north London, and for the first time read about the way I was behaving and why that might be (Perls 1968). That book helped me to develop some crucial personal insight. It was one of my biggest 'turn to moments', even if with a book rather than a person. Good personalised services depend upon a deep connection between the vulnerable individual and their supporters. Inevitably this has resource implications.

Personalisation as a paradigm has been enhanced by the citizen rights agenda. Posts such as the Children's Commissioners in England, Scotland Wales and Northern Ireland: posts of Children's Rights Directors and user champions within organisations, more recently, the appointment of a Commissioner for Older People in Wales; and frequent calls to extend the guardian role, currently only available for children in care, to vulnerable groups such as especially vulnerable older people and unaccompanied asylum seeking young people, all strengthen the focus on the needs, wishes, feelings and rights of individuals (see the International Guardianship Network at www.international-guardianship.com).

Despite consumerism and personalisation, 'the individual is always living some larger narrative, whether he or she likes it or not' (Stuart Hall, quoted in an interview for *The Observer Review*, 23 September 2007). There has to be a limit to personalisation, which is a form of partnership working between the individual, civic society and the state, well summed up as the balance between rights and responsibilities, and played out in continuing political scuffles about whether vulnerable people who use services could really hold down a job if they were forced to, or if any perverse incentives to stay off work were removed.

Partnership working and globalisation

The incremental impact of globalisation is massive and incalculable. 'Since the 1960s, the accelerating advance of globalisation, that is to say the world as a single unit of inter-connected activities unhampered by local boundaries, has had a profound political and cultural impact, especially in its currently dominant form of an uncontrolled global market' (Hobsbawm 2007).

Children in the UK now learn Mandarin as a main language, often in preference to German. Many Chinese families, with only one child as a consequence of the limits on family size, invest all their earnings in the education of their child. Some UK schools like Dulwich College have opened new schools in Shanghai to capitalise on this investment. Chinese and Indian social workers are now working in the UK, whilst their UK counterparts struggle to move the other way because of poorer language skills. In general terms, we are in a de-restricting era, with increasing traffic of all sorts across boundaries that were previously fixed or impenetrable. This brings opportunities as well as more risks like child trafficking. Some social problems, like teenage binge drinking, are as much a problem and concern in Australia as they are in the UK.

Inevitably, globalisation affects social care staff in their everyday work. The main family links for some children and families or vulnerable adults may be on another continent. Staff may be working with unaccompanied asylum-seeking children, or with illegal immigrants who become highly vulnerable and whose eligibility for the help they need is in question. A social care team may contain staff from many countries who are in the UK either temporarily or who may already have resettled, having worked in social care both outside and inside the UK. The social care task now includes selecting the best diversity framework to use in assessment and care planning. Social care training courses now include a requirement to understand international perspectives and cross-cultural competencies (Lyons 2006). As Lyons says:

> We must now think in terms of trans-national as well as trans-cultural social work and should aim for further developments in social work education and research to support social workers and service users. We are all now operating in – or struggling with – conditions affected by globalisation.

Care is also becoming internationalised as a result of the general easing of boundaries and less territorial approaches. Kent County Council forged partnerships with the United States for the recruitment of social workers and a knowledge exchange, and also placed older people in French residential care homes at a lower cost than they could purchase in Kent. In a similar vein, Norway builds and runs care and rehabilitation homes on the Spanish east coast on health as well as cost grounds.

Many UK councils now have partnerships with academic institutions and employers overseas for recruitment purposes – sometimes in defiance of the Savannah Accord, which is a pledge by nations not to poach each other's staff – and knowledge exchanges, which allow for useful international and cross-cultural lessons to be learnt and, where possible, applied. For example, in Switzerland, drugs policy is health-led rather than justice-led. Heroin is prescribed for drug users, reducing users' need to fund their habit through acquisitive crime. Switzerland has a lower burglary rate as a result. In the Netherlands, young social care workers caring for children have been redesignated as worker/carers, and are funded for meeting a caring need in their own family if and when it arises (Lewis 2006). This approach could help with social care recruitment and retention problems.

Globalisation brings with it risks, especially for complacent commissioners and providers. Venture capitalists have always had their eyes on potentially lucrative care markets and have acquired a number of private care companies, perhaps leading to a greater risk of asset stripping and loss of local control in the future.

At the community level, global partnerships are increasing. One is the partnership between tea growers in the Nilgiri Hills in Southern India and residents of the Marsh Farm Estate in North Luton, as part of a Fair Trade partnership (*The Guardian*, Society supplement, 12 September 2007). Another is the Glimmer of Hope Foundation. This funds projects in Ethiopia and UK inner cities, in a set of trans-national partnerships focusing on combating poverty and exclusion wherever they exist. It is funded by City traders wanting to put something back (www.aglimmerofhope.org). Other programmes like collaborative land-use management show the importance of community partnerships, most of which share the core social care principles and ideals.

The service equivalent of globalisation is eclecticism. This means in terms of theory, and applying theory to social care practice, that no single theoretical model will have a universal application. In a complex diverse society like the UK, the aim of a social care intervention will be to apply the right mix and combination of the various methods and theories available to each individual situation. This fusion model was adopted by the States of Guernsey Government, when determining a new family justice system in 2006. They decided to fuse the Scottish legal system with the English children's guardian model in Cafcass, producing a hybrid system which best suited their local circumstances.

Partnership working and public policy: the relationship between the individual, civic society and government

Towards a new political synthesis

In general, the project of government is to promote or sponsor a better society. Government has to add value to what economic circumstances produce of their own accord. Citizens have always thought of governments as being good, bad, or a necessary evil. In Siena, in 1377, the council commissioned Ambrogio Lorenzetti to decorate their council chamber. The cabinet members wanted the frescoes in the council chamber of the day to emphasise their underlying political convictions. The fresco to the right portrayed Bad Government, in the shape of a tyrant with devil-like features symbolising fear and oppression. The fresco to the left portrayed Good Government, showing people living in harmony with the state promoting by its actions the common good, security and wealth. Good contemporary government is not really that much different 600 years later. The role of the state is fairly fixed, despite short-term political turmoil. Any new government inherits a vast meta-system whose work is dictated by thousands of laws, regulation and working practices, and where operational accountability is shared uneasily between central, regional and local agencies.

A new government can only make minimal changes, hence it will always want to make those changes sound and seem far reaching. More recently, especially with globalisation and technological change, governments are simultaneously more aware of their own limitations, and of the need to work in a closer partnership with institutions in the broader civic society and with individuals themselves, who cannot be relied upon or corralled as easily as they once could be. As a result, 'a new political synthesis' is being sought by politicians and highlighted by political theorists (Williamson *et al.* 2003). I referred above to one example: a future partnership between citizens and the state about the funding of personal care, implying a new social contract, with a redefinition of the respective responsibilities of government and citizens. Another is the development of an asset-based partnership scheme, with proposals for the state to provide citizens with greater incentives to save, through Partnership Savings schemes (Le Grand 2003). UK courts have witnessed a mini-explosion of people representing themselves in all sorts of hearings, as litigants-in-person. The state and individual citizens are constantly redefining themselves and their inter-relationship.

Critics still see the state in terms of either being too nanny-like or too neglectful, whilst public expectations grow all the time. 'There is growing awareness of how difficult it is for governments to meet the expectations of an increasingly affluent and discriminating electorate. Citizens expect high quality services and the definition of "high quality" is rising all the time' (Kelly 2000). Politicians have recently been buffeted by another mini-explosion, this time of single-issue pressure groups, with campaigns conducted over the internet using YouTube or other media to get their message across to a large audience in an instant, and with extensions to local democracy such as the right of 250 people signing a petition to force their local council to consider any proposal. With new media, no permission is needed to get your message across. As Miranda Lewis says, 'Policy is moving towards a sense of partnership between state and citizen which aims to ensure that people are empowered to solve problems themselves, and away from a situation in which decisions are taken on our behalf' (Lewis 2007).

Place shaping

'Place shaping' is the way in which government, through local partnerships, aims to mould the UK, its regions, subregions and local areas, to meet the

Shaping Burnley

Community tensions increased in the 1990s because of the changing face of the town, culminating in street riots in 2001. The cotton industry and a large Irish immigrant community (Central Station was known as the Irish Park), gave way to engineering firms and immigration by people with a Pakistani heritage into North Burnley. Stoneyholme with Daneshouse, the ward with the highest proportion of people of Asian residents, has the highest birth rate, more than double the rate in wards like Cliviger with Worsthorne. These statistics are borne out nationally. Working Pakistani and Bangladeshi households are more likely to be in poverty than workless white households (Department for Work and Pensions).

Action groups in Burnley include the Burnley Action Partnership, Burnley Youth Council, Building Bridges in Burnley (an interfaith organisation), and groups working to stage the annual Burnley Community Festival. The Burnley Action Partnership aims to reduce segregation – particularly a predominant housing and educational segregation – and, with it, the resulting tensions and polarisation. As a result of their work, the percentage of people from different backgrounds who feel that their local area is a place where they can get on well together, rose from 35 per cent in 2003 to 48 per cent in 2005 (*The Real Story*, Burnley Borough Council 2006). Integration programmes continue, including major new school building programmes. One site, on the periphery of Stoneyholme with Daneshouse, includes a faith centre to promote integration and equality.

Key place-shaping questions across the UK are:

- What is my town becoming?
- What is my street becoming?
- What is my village becoming?
- What is my country becoming?

Burnley's experience and problem solving is being repeated in every local community affected by social change in the UK.

changing demographics and expectations I have described earlier in this chapter. The increasing political priority attached to place shaping is due to findings such as a MORI poll in 2007 which reported that 50 per cent of Britons believe that we run the real risk of a divided society if we don't redefine what Britishness means. A message on a kiosk from Birmingham City Council to passers-by in the city centre proclaims: 'United Streets of Birmingham: these are our streets, let's look out for them'. The strong message from government, in several key reports like the Cantle report (Cantle 2001) is about increasing and improving partnership working between communities through greater 'community cohesion', between local agencies and local communities – indeed, through every partnership combination imaginable, in order to limit any negative impact of rapid social change.

Local areas and communities are changing fast. In the Bangladeshi community in Tower Hamlets, many local residents are pooling their resources to support children in after school classes, building up social capital and a stronger civil society in the process. Change tends to be faster in immigrant communities, who often have to act more quickly to establish themselves. The negative press about immigration is often countered by a relative ease of assimilation in some towns and cities. The 22,000 Poles in Slough live relatively harmoniously, placing little burden upon local services (Rose 2008). However, it is impossible to generalise about integration, especially about which communities will and won't or can and can't integrate. In colliery villages like Wath near Barnsley in South Yorkshire, the Barnsley of Kes, Billy Elliott and Dickie Bird, some families, whose male breadwinners were on opposite sides in the miner's dispute over 20 years ago, are still not talking to each other.

Arguably, one role of government is to reduce dependency upon the state and to promote broader forms of asset ownership. Seventy-five per cent of wealth in some communities is public-sector money. The public sector is still the largest employer in many towns and cities in the UK. For example, in Leeds, the biggest employers are Leeds City Council (35,000 staff), Leeds General Infirmary (15,000 staff) and the University of Leeds (8,000 staff), whereas the largest private sector employer is Asda with 1,000 staff. To respond to the pace and scale of change, public policy in relation to a specific town, city region or subregion needs to be co-ordinated. For example, the programme to close local post offices, bizarrely called the urban re-invention programme, failed to take into account the level of use, particularly in poor communities who are the highest users of postal services, because the programme was actually a 'strategic reshaping of the network based mainly on distance access criteria and sub-postmasters' preferences' (National Consumer Council 2007a).

Co-ordination in real time is rendered increasingly problematic by the sheer quantity and variety of phenomena acting upon a local place. Some local people have concerns that place shaping can become a form of class or community cleansing, with local people being ostracised and removed to create new property developments with a wealthier demographic. The difficulty of place shaping is illustrated in Salford, Greater Manchester, where the council and developers encouraged people moving in to form a new community, but in fact many of those new residents brought major social problems in with them.

Place shaping includes improving public health through partnership working, as it has done for nearly 150 years since the construction of a universal clean water supply in UK cities dramatically reduced cholera

A state within: the complexity of place shaping

Whilst many people living in the UK feel a degree of detachment from the way the country is run, and from local civil society, some groups go further and form a state within the state, with different values and a strong internal support system.

For example, young Muslim girls wishing to rebel against a forced marriage, or other traditional and often tribal structures brought over wholesale into the UK from the subcontinent, may only be able to leave by joining a radical fundamentalist group who offer an alternative support structure which may involve up to 100 women being mobilised to support a single girl or young woman in conflict with her extended family (Malik 2007). At present, UK society and institutions have little to offer alienated young Asians who feel that 'this mixed heritage of being British by birth, Asian by descent and Muslim by conviction, was set to tear me apart in later life' (Husain 2007). Many partnerships are based upon one partner offering a refuge or safe haven to someone determined to escape from a situation, family or culture they find stultifying.

The state has to find ways of supporting alienated youth with an alternative identity, if the individual and social problems experienced by these young people, and the social and personal difficulties they can experience and create as a result, are to be reduced and ultimately avoided.

outbreaks. In Vermont, USA, between 1994 and 1999, elevated blood levels of lead in local people, caused by lead paint in house-building, fell from 11.3 per cent to 3.3 per cent as a result of sustained action by the local council to renovate its older housing stock (McCauley and Cleaver 2006). Today's social and health concerns, like violent crime and obesity, all require sustained partnership working programmes, relevant to each community and each 'place'.

The potential for partnership working, through various state-sponsored processes, to regenerate an area for the benefit of the next generation is clear, but 'the strength of embedded behaviours and cultures should not be underestimated (Wistow 2007).

The language of partnerships

Use of the word *partnership* is itself an indicator of its significance. In 1989, the word was used in parliament 38 times, but by 1999, this had increased to 6,197 times (Jup 2000).

Transforming Shoreditch

My second social work job was in Shoreditch, between 1976 and 1978, working in a substandard office in a run-down part of East London. The office I worked in, the adjacent DHSS local office and a woodyard importing exotic hardwoods which I used to equip my family's kitchen at the time, have all long gone, to be replaced by a JobCentrePlus – the DHHS office upgraded or at least renamed – and a new community college.

The Shoreditch Trust, a New Deal for Communities Project (NDC), has delivered a series of regeneration initiatives, originally sponsored to the tune of £60 million over ten years by Renaisi, the Hackney Council development agency for regeneration programmes throughout the London borough. To some extent Shoreditch was in the right place at the right time – on the northern fringe of the City of London, when the city was ripe for expansion. The area is now filled with new environmentally friendly restaurants, bars and small businesses, and developments are co-ordinated by the trust and its community-led board. Educational results are better, employment is better and crime has been reduced. The housing stock has proved harder to transform, and the 'credit crunch' in 2008 may make this element of the regeneration programme difficult for a generation to come.

Hackney Council seconded me to become a qualified social worker and I worked there for 12 years, for seven years as a social worker, and then eight years later as an Assistant Director of Social Services for five years. They were personally formative times. I was one of many thousands of people whose living or working lives were changed for the better by working in and around Shoreditch. We helped to shape the place, and the place helped to shape us.

If, as the urban myth would have it, eskimos have more than 50 words for snow, ' partnership working' is not far behind. Terms such as 'co-production', in which the service user plays an equally active role to the professional worker, 'blended families', connected care and 'hybridisation', are starting to enter the partnership lexicon (Mottiar and White 2003). With language, an element of free extension is inevitable. The department stores, John Lewis and Waitrose, have a partnership card which functions as a storecard and a credit card. Can a credit card really be thought of as a partnership? They would say yes – their staff are associates and partners, and like all retailers they wish to attract a loyal customer base who think of themselves as in a personal retail partnership with the stores. Language is free of course and has always been colonised and adapted. It is also a fact of life that a new study coins new terms to draw attention to itself. For example, we should build 'a constituency of concern' (user voices), with 'differentiated consumers' (they're all different) according to the National Consumer Council in their study *OurSay: User Voice and Public Service Culture* (National Consumer Council 2007b).

Language is being inflated and managerialised, erecting ladders of abstraction. So tourism has become destination management. A market is now an economic development centre. Finishing a project is execution management. Accident and Emergency Departments are becoming Urgent Care Centres. Large GP surgeries providing day surgery are becoming polyclinics. 'Reticulists' (Murphy 1996) are individuals committed to change who act as 'entrepreneurs of power' (Degeling 1995). 'Boundary spanners' are partnership co-ordinators who iron out problems, sometimes known as 'organisational operators' (Thompson 2003). 'Flexicurity' denotes flexible but secure workplaces. For management consultants, SMEs are crucial – subject matter experts. Jargon is distancing – 'the complex and specialist terminologies used often vary between agencies and can be difficult for parents, or indeed for other professionals, to understand (Boddy *et al.* 2006).

Using a simple shared language can assist in the consolidation of partnership working, particularly the use of shared narratives to describe the common situations faced by professionals. Language can convey the values underpinning a partnership and partnership 'keywords' include trust, betrayal and loyalty as much as technical jargon. Language can also be memorable and define a profession's values. When Baroness Elizabeth Butler Sloss, in the Cleveland Inquiry report, said that 'the child is a person and not an object of concern', that phrase came to inspirationally symbolise child-centred social work for thousands of social workers. A roundabout I saw in India had two words repeated around its circumference: compassion and kindness. A bridge in Rochdale, England, has 'the birthplace of co-operation' painted across it, signifying the start of the co-operative movement in the UK – a value-laden message. Context and geography are also important elements of social care language. In Scottish family law cases, those bringing and defending cases are known as pursuers and defenders respectively, whilst in England they are called applicants and respondents. The threshold for being defined as 'old' in respect of eligibility for services, is 60, 65, 75 or 80, depending on the nature of the service and the policies of the provider.

Language that inspires, language that depresses

The language of social care has become a hard and bureaucratic dialect. Assessments, care plans, allocation – all are uninspiring managerial words, however necessary. Yet according to Evans *et al.* (2007) 'Choice of language can help to dictate the climate and culture in which services are provided'. Two relatively new concepts, resilience and forgiveness, are examples of language which practitioners and people who use services can engage with more. Resilience is a term with applications for everyone involved in a social

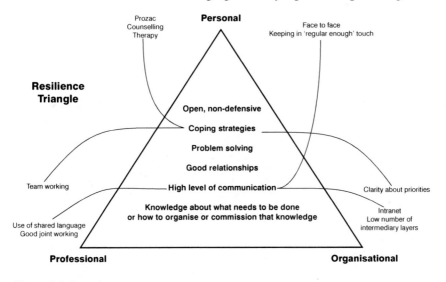

Figure 2.1 Capacity

care network. People who use services, staff and organisations need to develop resilience to cope with adverse circumstances (see Figure 2.2 and 'Beyond language' box). Forgiveness is an underused word in working with people who use services, staff and, once again, organisations. Children frequently forgive their parents for poor standards of care, and this is relevant in work to reunify children with their parents. Staff make mistakes and usually need to be forgiven rather than harangued. Organisations need to learn the art of forgiveness, but rarely see themselves as operating in the world of emotional intelligence they in reality inhabit.

As well as values, culture shifts can also be expressed by changing a single word or phrase. The move from 'clients' to 'people who use services' and 'service integrators', are word shifts symbolising a profound culture change for people who use services from a status of passive recipient to actively engaged and empowered partner. The change in title from the Waifs and Strays Society (1881), to the Church of England Children's Society (1946), and, since 1982, the Children's Society, is another example of the need to update language to reflect the times even if the underlying values and motivation remain the same. When some carers groups renamed themselves as family carers groups, their membership shot up, because family carers instantly realised this referred to them, whereas references to unpaid carers or informal carers, still used by many groups, passed them by.

With any culture shift, the language associated with that shift can be muddled, and practitioners still lack a simple shared terminology even for their clients. 'Over the last fifty years, the discourse in Britain about 'racialised minorities' has mutated from 'colour' in the 1950s and 1960s ... to 'race' in the 1960s, 1970s and 1980s ... to 'ethnicity' in the 1990s ... and to

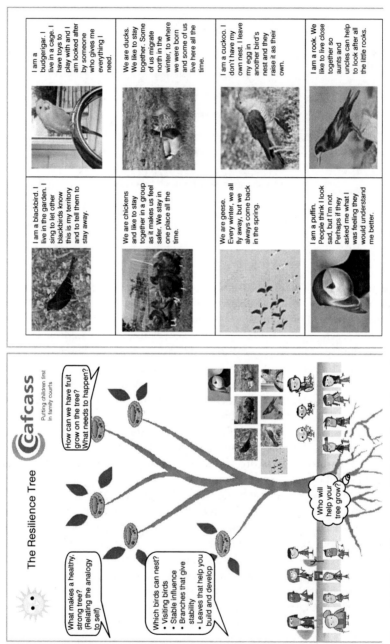

Figure 2.2 The resilience tree. Which bird would you choose to live in your tree?

Beyond language: 'the resilience tree'

The resilience tree is a tool for social care staff to communicate with young children for whom language is difficult, and where a more visual and emotional language is needed to support effective interaction and communication. This and similar tools support partnership working where conventional language doesn't work – more than 50 per cent of children who come into care through family court applications are under six years old, so tools like this are essential. The fact that over 90 per cent of communication between two people is non-verbal, and less than 10 per cent is verbal, shows why communication tools support effective partnership working between people who use services and professionals.

Language in action: job descriptions

Traditional job descriptions for staff tend to list the main duties and responsibilities that an employee has to undertake and then the personal characteristics they must have to be ready, willing and able to be successful. To assist partnership working, a greater focus on the outcomes of either a single agency post or a joint post, and how those can be achieved by working with others, can support partnership working by providing a stronger linguistic and conceptual framework for staff to understand what is required of them.

A social worker's job description might have been: 'under the line management of the service manager, to provide social work advice and support across all services for people with sensory impairment' and 'by agreement with the relevant team manager, to undertake ongoing care management in certain identified cases'. A more outcome-focused job description might say: 'to ensure that advice and support to people who use services helps to improve their situation', and 'to ensure the care received by people on your caseload is of the highest quality and is freely chosen, taking into account any professional assessments'.

'religion' in the present time (Beckford *et al.* 2006). Similarly, the English Children's Commissioner's Office was renamed in 2006 as '11 million' – the number of children in England.

This rebranding, aiming for greater impact and public awareness, shows the importance of name recognition to organisations – the NSPCC is recognised by over 70 per cent of the UK population, whereas recognition for some other leading charities is under 30 per cent. Rebranding is also undertaken to emphasise a change in values. For example, the government now refers to the teaching profession as the learning profession, attempting by changing a single word to describe a culture shift. An image can change quickly: the NSPCC was known as 'the cruelty' until the 1980s, and some of its inspectors continued to wear uniforms until that time. A smaller number remained in tied (to employment) accommodation until well into the 1990s. This illustrates how a new image for an organisation in the outside world often runs decades ahead of changes in working practices inside that same organisation.

Language can also help to shape values such as dignity. 'Backward – "why don't they just call them backward?" Everyone knows what it means' or 'she's a mongol'. These are derogatory terms: 'people with learning difficulties' is less derogatory, but referring to people, whatever their difficulties, with their name, in the same way everyone else is referred to, is the requisite language of dignity.

Communication is not always straightforward or obvious. Clichés that slip into common use can be misleading. When described as 'hard to reach', many young people's groups say, 'we're not hard to reach, you're just bad at reaching us!'

Words and language do matter. Many words written by social care professionals are pored over, usually retrospectively and with the benefit of hindsight, for example in complaints investigations. Freedom of information (FOI) legislation also means it is best if professionals assume everything they say and write down could be the subject of an application to see it under FOI. At worst, this encourages defensive practice – deleting emails and shredding papers once they have been used. At best, the trend towards openness will bring greater accountability in the use of language and what is being expressed, to promote stronger and more open partnerships, including a stronger 'vocabulary of collaboration' (Integrated Care Network 2008).

References

Beckett, F., 1997, *Clem Attlee*, London: Richard Cohen Books.

Beckford, A., Gayle, R., Owen, D., Peach, C. and Weller, P., 2006, *Review of the Evidence Base on Faith Communities*, quoted in J. Boddy, P. Potts and J. Statham, 2006, *Models of Good Practice in Joined-Up Assessment: Working for Children with Significant and Complex Needs*, London: Thomas Coram Research Unit.

Cantle, T., 2001, *Community Cohesion*, London: Home Office.

CSCI, 2008, *The State of Social Care in England*, London: CSCI.

CSCI, GSCC and SCIE, 2007, *Facing the Facts: Social Care in England*, London: CSCI.

Degeling, P., 1995, 'The significance of "sectors" in calls for urban public health: intersectoralism: an Australian perspective', *Policy and Politics*, 23(4): 289–301.

Department of Health, 2001, *Valuing People: A New Strategy for Learning Disabilities for the 21st Century*, London: Department of Health.

Department of Health, 2006, *Our Health, Our Care, Our Say: A New Direction for Community Services*, London: Department of Health.

Department of Health, 2008, *Seven Common Core Principles to Support Self Care*, London: NHS (available at: www.networks.nhs.uk/news.php?nid=2213).

Donaghy, C. and McReynolds, F., 2004, 'Building effective cross-border co-operation in health and social services in the border regions of Ireland', paper given at the European Social Services Conference, Dublin, 20 June.

Duffy, S., 2008, *Ethical Values: The Beliefs and Values That Underpin In Control's Work*, Birmingham: In Control.

Evans, I., Yamaguchi, T., Raskauskas, J. and Harvey, S., 2007, *Fairness, Forgiveness and Families*, Wellington: New Zealand Families Commission.

Gibbons, B., 2007, 'Devolution in practice: health policy', *New Statesman*, 29 January.

Gilbert, P., 2007, 'Engaging hearts and minds – and the spirit', *Journal of Integrated Care*, 15(4): 11, 20–6.

Goldson, J., 2006, *Hello, I'm a Voice, Let Me Talk: Child Inclusive Mediation in Family Separation*, Wellington: New Zealand Families Commission.

Ham, C., 2004, *Health Policy in Britain*, Basingstoke: Palgrave.

Henwood, M. and Hudson, B., 2007, *Here to Stay? Self-Directed Support: Aspiration and Implementation*, a review for the Department of Health, London: Department of Health.

Hall, S., 2007, quoted in 'Cultural Hallmark', *The Observer*, 23 September.

HM Government, 2007, *Putting People First: A Shared Vision and Commitment to the Transformation of Adult Social Care*, London: HM Government.

Hobsbawm, E., 2007, *Globalisation, Democracy and Terrorism*, New York: Little, Brown.

Hudson, B., 2007, 'Partnering through networks: can Scotland crack it?,' *Journal of Integrated Care*, 15(1): 3–13.

Husain, E., 2007, *The Islamist*, Harmondsworth: Penguin Books.

Integrated Care Network, 2008, *Bringing the NHS and Local Government Together: A Practical Guide to Integrated Working*, London: Integrated Care Network (as part of the Care Services Improvement Partnership, Department of Health).

Jordan, B., 2006, Review of 'well-being: the next revolution in children's services', *Journal of Children's Services*, 1(1): 41–50.

Jupp, B., 2000, *Working Together: Creating a Better Environment for Cross-Sector Partnerships*, London: Demos.

Kelly, G., 2000, *The New Partnership Agenda*, London: IPPR.

Kerr, D., 2005, *Building a Health Service Fit for the Future: A Report on the Future of the NHS in Scotland*, Edinburgh: Scottish Executive.

Kerr, M., 2004, 'Improving the general health of people with learning disabilities', *Advances in Psychiatric Treatment*, 10(2): 200–6.

Le Grand, J., 2003, *Motivation, Agency and Public Policy*, Oxford: Oxford University Press.

Lewis, J., 2006, 'Care and gender: have the arguments for recognising care work now been won?', in C. Glendinning and P. Kemp (eds), *Cash and Care: Policy Challenges in the Welfare State*, Bristol: Policy Press.

Lewis, M., 2007, 'From the public to the private sphere', in *Regulating Right: Regulation Shows Its Better and Local Faces*, Portland, OR: Solace Foundation.

LGA, 2006, *Without a Care?* London: LGA.

LGA, 2008, *Prosperous Communities 11: Vive la Dévolution!*, London: LGA.

Lyons, K., 2006, 'Globalisation and social work: international and local implications', *British Journal of Social Work*, 36(3): 365–80.

Malik, S., 2007, 'The making of a terrorist', *Prospect Magazine*, June.

Martin, E. and Law, J., 2006, *Oxford Dictionary of Law*, Oxford: Oxford University Press.

McCauley, C. and Cleaver, D., 2006, *Improving Service Delivery: Introducing Outcomes-based Accountability*, London: IdeA.

Mottiar, S. and White, F., 2003, *Co-production as a Form of Service Delivery*, Johannesburg: Centre for Policy Studies.

Mencap, 2003, *Out of Sight, Out of Mind*, London: Mencap.

Murphy, M., 1996, *The Child Protection Unit*, London: Ashgate.

National Consumer Council, 2007a, *Post Office Closures 2002 to 2006: Lessons for 2007 to 2009*, London: National Consumer Council.

National Consumer Council, 2007b, *Our Say: User Voice and Public Service Culture*, London: National Consumer Council.

Parsons, T., 2008, *My Favourite Wife*, New York: HarperCollins.

Perls, F., 1968, *Ego, Hunger and Aggression*, London: Vintage Books.

Pugh, G., 2007, *London's Forgotten Children*, Stroud: Tempus.

Social Exclusion Unit, 2006, *Reaching Out: An Action Plan on Social Exclusion*, London: Social Exclusion Unit.

Rhodes, R.A.W., 1997, *Understanding Governance: Policy Networks, Governance, Reflexivity and Accountability*, Oxford: Oxford University Press.

Rose, D., 2006, 'How migrants fuel Britain's boom town', *The Observer*, 6 April.

Thompson, W.D., 2003, *Organizations in Action: Social Science Bases of Administrative Theory*, new edn, Piscataway, NJ: Transaction Publishers.

Varney, D., 2006, *Public Service Transformation Review*, London: HM Treasury.

Wanless, D., 2004, *Securing Good Health for the Whole Population*, London: HM Treasury.

Wanless, D., 2006, *Securing Good Care for Older People: Taking a Long-term View*, London: HM Treasury.

Weatherburn, P., Keogh, P., Dodds, C., Hickson, F. and Henderson, L., 2007, *The Growing Challenge: A Strategic Review of HIV Social Care, Support and Information Services Across the UK*, London: Aids Funders Forum.

Williamson, T., Imbroscio, D. and Alperovitz, G., 2003, *Making a Place for Community*, Oxon: Routledge.

Wistow, G., 2007, 'Successful governance is all in the mix', in *Loose Talk and a Hard Nut: Commissioning for Better Outcomes*, Portland, OR: Solace Foundation.

3   Who are the partners?

Part 1: Social care partnerships

Key messages

- The major partnership in social care is with those who use its services – this partnership is turning social care on its head.
- Partnerships with carers need to ensure that all carers have a support system
- Joint working between professional groups is no easier than it was 20 years ago, and wholesale structural change is likely to weaken links rather than strengthen them – concentrating on improving and supporting joint working is better
- Some intractable problems, such as inequality of access to services and marginalisation, do not automatically improve with partnership working – at most it is a better framework

---

Partnerships with people who use services

> He aha te mea nui o tenei ao maku e ki atu. He tangata! He tangata! He tangata! [Ask me what is most important in this world. Let me tell you. It is people! It is people! It is people!]
>
> (Maori proverb)

> I must have been at the heart of it (my case) because I had a care order made, but I was never part of it.
>
> (Jerome 2007)

The transformation in partnership culture under way

The key partnership in twenty-first-century social care is between organisations and those who use their services – partnership working as a process between professionals and people who use services, not as new structures or new organisations. The transformation in culture required can be illustrated by the words of an abuse survivor, who said 'I don't think I've got emotions about anything now' (speaking on the Today programme, 29 February 2008). He was speaking some 30 years after allegedly being abused in a Jersey children's home, Haut de la Garenne, where acts of torture and abuse reminiscent of earlier centuries were allegedly committed. These acts – impossible to speak about at the time – were mirrored elsewhere in the UK such as North Wales (Waterhouse 2000), and abroad in institutions like the Catholic church in Ireland (Ridge 2008).

The risks of abusive cultures, in total or closed institutions, remain high to this day, so shielded are they from external scrutiny on a day-to day-basis, and so controlling are the internal working cultures for residents and staff. To combat depersonalisation of prisoners, a former Director General of the Prison Service instructed that by Day 6 of their admission, every new prisoner would be addressed as Mister or by their first name, in an attempt to humanise prison culture and develop a sense of partnership between prison officers and their prisoners.

The contrast between these punitive cultures and the person-centred service that some people now receive is stark. The care package for one adult service user in Oldham today includes a season ticket to Blackburn Rovers and respite care in Tenerife. In one scenario a service user is nearly obliterated, in the other, the service user is treated equally and democratically – a process which can be described as 'putting service users into the middle of the organisation', as 'experts in their own experience'. This can include service users, including looked-after children, chairing their own statutory review meetings with support to do so, or generating and shaping the content of websites which offer support advice and information to service user groups (Watson 2008).

Such respect-based services need to be 'mainstreamed', in processes such as joint recording rather than service users not being aware of what has been written about them. The quality of service received should also not be a function of where you live, or who your care worker happens to be, as it is now. As Blaise Pascal said, 'the strength of a man's virtue must not be measured by his occasional efforts but by his ordinary life' (Pascal 1669).

Many professional staff need to go though a sea change in attitude and mind-set to 'work together' with people who use services. This can be equated with treating people who user services as you would a close friend. As a newly qualified social worker, in 1980, I needed to assess the risks an elderly demented woman posed to herself in her own flat. Neighbours said she left the gas on and wandered out into the street in her nightclothes, leaving her television blaring all night. Nowadays, I would not be a generic social worker, trying to do everything, but a community care worker, almost certainly more experienced in assessing the needs of older people with dementia. Given those skills, I would look first at support options in the community. But in 1980, I asked my team manager, who was close to retirement, what I should do.

Joint review of AB: professionals and relatives reviewing together

When a mental health patient dies, an NHS Serious Incident Inquiry has to be convened. In the case of the death of a young man (AB) suffering from schizophrenia, the review was co-produced by Sherrie Hitchen, in collaboration with the family members of AB, in order to fully reflect the family's perspective. The process concentrated on the collaborative process of writing the review, particularly 'agreeing the facts and conclusions in an ethos of shared knowledge and understanding' (Hitchen 2007). 'The process of writing reports in this collaborative style is slow, and can be emotionally painful and challenging for relatives, and to a lesser extent, for the report authors' (ibid.). The payoff is invariably a greater understanding by family survivors of how and why an event like this happened, often enabling a degree of resolution and closure.

This way of working has innumerable extensions in daily professional life throughout social care services. It can be contrasted with the tokenistic inclusion of service users in processes and structures they find impossible to relate to:

> professionals seek to draw service users into their pre-existing professional structures and systems with little regard for whether such systems (usually formal meetings and loads of paperwork) are actually appropriate or relevant to the users with whom they are trying to work. Whilst some users may find these systems useful, others know that they are not for them or have learned by bitter experience how disempowering, intimidating and emotionally battering they can be, especially for those who have been most disadvantaged by the system.
>
> (Trivedi 2002)

The key principle to observe is that 'instead of professionals being in the driving seat, service users and professionals travel together' (Begum 2006). An example of empowerment in practice, is that if disabled people do come to meetings to 'participate', this is counted as 'committed work' in relation to any statutory benefits they receive.

Much partnership working with service users, especially as members of boards or committees within governance structures, has been condemned as tokenistic but as Peck and Glasby observe, 'it is perhaps unhelpful to ... use the pejorative term "tokenistic", as this seems to both impute the motives of the organisation and deny the wider implications of their membership' (Peck and Glasby 2004). Whilst there is rarely an intention to subject people who use services to another level of marginalisation, it is very often the unintended consequence.

Matter of factly, she said: 'She needs to be in the German Hospital [the local psychiatric unit, or mental hospital as it was called then]. Just tell her she's going on holiday, then bring her round to the back door of the office. I'll have an ambulance waiting.' I am ashamed to say I did. It took me another eight years to realise that the people who mattered most in service provision were those on the receiving end!

Getting alongside service users

'What did you do to make people listen to you when you said you didn't want to stay at your foster carers?' 'I set their house on fire'.
(a boy in care – story told to me by
Professor Adrian James from Sheffield University)

Why build a chocolate wall in your mother's bedroom?
(a social care practitioner speaking to a man with learning disabilities
still living at home – the chocolate wall had meaning for him)

Soochne ke bimaari … my sorrow has become my illness.
(Asian woman after visiting her English doctor, cited in CRE 1999)

These three quotes illustrate the power of the service user experience and behaviour, and the extent of the adaptation required by many professionals to get alongside vulnerable children and adults experiencing considerable distress, particularly those without speech, or who speak a different language, or who are too young or distressed to express themselves. The situations that people who use services find themselves in can sometimes mean that saying nothing, or flatly denying a problem, is a rational act. As Albert Camus would have said in his seminal novel about alienation, *The Outsider*, 'many parents in care proceedings are "outsiders at their own party", looking on blankly and non-committally as professionals decide their fate' (Camus 1942). The inability to speak out, either through a disability, through not being able to speak English, or emotional withdrawal, places people who need services at a higher level of risk than normal. Two per cent of disabled children in need are on English child protection registers compared with eight per cent of the general population of children in need (Cooke 2000). Concerns about the abuse of disabled children are 50 per cent less likely to be case conferenced – see Table 3.1 (Cooke and Standen 2002).

Understanding and engaging with different groups of service users lies at the heart of good joint working. Working with a Sikh family will need a basic knowledge of Sikhism. Gender-sensitive services require an understanding of how to deliver effective services to vulnerable men and women. Policy and campaigning groups like Fathers Direct recommend agencies carry out a 'male involvement audit', to see how many male service users, volunteers and staff they have, and ask 'what part are they playing in planning, implementing,

Table 3.1 Likelihood of abuse of disabled children

Type of maltreatment	Crosse et al. (1993)	Sullivan and Knutson (1997, 2000)
Neglect	1.6 times as likely	3.8 times as likely
Sexual abuse	1.8 times as likely	3.1 times as likely
Physical abuse	2.1 times as likely	3.8 times as likely
Emotional maltreatment	2.8 times as likely	3.9 times as likely

monitoring and evaluating services?' (Fathers Direct 2005). *Peace of Mind*, a parenting course for Somali fathers in north London, run by Fathers Direct, aims at confidence-building after trauma and illustrates the importance of confidence and capacity-building in partnership working with service users. The sum total of these service-user-centric developments is that more people who need services are likely to find someone to represent their 'voice'. For example, Victim's Voice supports victims of crime to express themselves in court and are working with the Ministry of Justice to pilot a Victim's Advocate scheme – another vulnerable group starting to receive support from a State-funded organisation at their lowest point.

Two-way communication

Communication, with service users and professionals, should always be checked to ensure understanding is mutual (Reder and Duncan 2006). Communicating under pressure can cause meaning to be lost in translation. When Tony Blair met the French Socialist leader Lionel Jospin, he gave a speech in French and was so over-confident he decided to answer journalists in French too. His response to one question, when he said he admired Jospin's stance on many policy issues, was translated as 'I desire him in many positions'!

Social care professionals and people who need services often meet under fraught circumstances – imagine you are a 10-year-old girl where there is a suspicion you have been sexually abused, and in the nicest possible way, a social worker, perhaps jointly with a police officer, asks you about this. If the barriers between professionals are sometimes towering, then think of how high the barriers between people who use services and professionals can be.

People who use services value those professionals who show emotion and come across as a real person who cares about them. 'Children and young people value practitioners who enjoy working with them, who treat them with respect and who are good at communicating with them' (GSCC 2007). The importance of making a positive personal impact is true whether the social work task is counselling or an assessment of need. Working professionally and behaving responsibly is one of the GSCC's core requirements of social workers' professional standards (and all social care professionals in the future). The individual social worker's partnership with the GSCC as regulator of conduct

David Jones (2003) identifies the core skills and qualities for effective communication with vulnerable children as:

- listening to the child
- conveying genuine interest
- empathic concern
- understanding
- emotional warmth
- respect for the child
- capacity to manage and contain the assessment
- awareness of the entire transaction between interviewer and child
- self-management
- technique

and standards is increasingly important. Students undergoing training are being brought up in a much fuller knowledge of its codes of practice and requirements than practitioners in the field, who still too often see their re-registration with the GSCC as another bureaucratic chore.

A key 'rule of engagement' for professionals is to listen to people asking for a service, before pronouncing judgment. One Plus One, teaches brief counselling techniques to professionals like GPs who only have five to ten minutes with each patient, during which time they have to make a diagnosis. One Plus One teach that many GPs spend the first eight of the ten minutes talking 'at' a patient, whereas it is more effective spending the first seven or eight minutes listening, to accumulate enough information to make an informed judgement about what it means.

Being sensitive to people who use services starts before the first meeting. A group of young Muslim women working with Cafcass advise practitioners to 'not dress in a suit on your first meeting' and, 'when a young woman reaches a certain age, the gender of the practitioner is important. This is the same for young Muslim males. It would be good to discuss this with the young person and their parents' (Cafcass 2007). Other young people said to the NSPCC 'Don't go ahead [and investigate] without telling me what is happening' (12-year-old). 'I wouldn't want them to laugh or for them not to believe me' (10-year-old) – and another 10-year-old when asked how adults should work with young people said 'you need a relationship' (Timms *et al.* 2007).

Emotional authenticity

The key value in the relationship between service users and social care staff is honesty. Complete trust is unlikely and unwise due to the power imbalance and the real or perceived sense of personal liberty sometimes being at stake. But honesty must be taken for granted. My first mental health admission was

an unacceptable infringement of the human rights of the woman concerned. For a sense of partnership to be felt, emotional authenticity is vital. Social care workers have to use their personalities in order to make and sustain a professional relationship. The relationship can never be a partnership of equals, but it can be based on mutual respect. Whilst some social care services can be arranged efficiently through call centres without a relationship, even the assessment for the simplest level of service, such as a meals service, benefits from a professional assessor meeting and understanding an older person with severe mobility problems, or discussing their needs with a referring professional or relative with skill and sensitivity.

Service user engagement

This shift in the balance of power between professionals and people who use services is easier to develop if agencies already have a strong culture of participation and engagement. Such engagement has to be a core part of how a referral or case is handled, not just an afterthought or a number of quasi-artificial set pieces in which everyone involved merely goes through the motions. For example, in casework, a theory map is literally a map of the theories and knowledge base a professional draws from when she or he forms a judgement or makes a decision. This can be shown to service users either by an agency or an individual practitioner, so the basis for decision-making is transparent.

Involving service users in the work of an agency from top to bottom is another way of promoting culture change. This can entail involvement in the recruitment of senior staff, in training practitioners or as members of internal inspection and audit teams – as young inspectors. Ealing Council's Corporate Parent Committee is led by young people and chaired by the council leader. It focuses on the authority's 450 children in care and 225 care leavers. Over 12 per cent of care leavers go to university, well above the national average. Young people wanted more work experience, a demand which directly led to the development of an accredited young apprentice scheme. Involvement brings with it more likelihood of policy implementation. Despite massive publicity, the only schools which have made progress to date with healthy living menus at lunchtime are those where children themselves have been involved in deciding the menu options and table layout.

User-led services, user-defined services, user-commissioned services and self-assessment, are becoming more widespread, with the role for professional staff becoming essentially facilitative. For instance, in Queensland, Australia, couples seeking an inter-country adoption can compile their own files and send them directly to an overseas agency. In Big and Teen Safe Houses for 15–16-year-olds, hosted by the No Limits agency in Southampton, young people determine how the service is run.

People who use services are actively engaged in partnership working throughout Europe. In Bordeaux, France, a users committee was established to oversee all the city's social exclusion projects as a mainstream and long-term commitment to working in partnership. In the Haut-des-Seines in France, a peri-natal network supports pregnant women and mothers with babies at risk, drawing upon trained African 'relay women', part of whose focus is population integration. Dasln is a database of children with autism spectrum disorder living in the northeast of England, owned and developed collaboratively by parents in Sunderland, Newcastle, Gateshead and Northumberland.

However, the tension between the respective value systems of safeguarding and engagement, or protection and participation, is becoming a serious cause of policy confusion and tension in many social care agencies (Welbourne 2002). Other agencies say they are too busy to spend serious time on participation and engagement, and these agencies are likely to score poorly on feedback from service users about partnership working.

Service user stories

Service user stories can support other users going through similar experiences, and can help promote a strong service-user-centric culture inside organisations. They also illustrate why partnership working is important from the perspective of those who need and use services.

Asparagus Dreams, a book written about her life by Jessica Peers, who was diagnosed at 12 with Asperger's syndrome, is in a growing tradition of books, poems, blogs written by service users about how they cope and often survive vulnerability, YouTube videos, citizen journalism in all its forms, and the role of professional services in supporting them (Peers 2003). Libby Rees is a girl who has written two children's self-help books by the age of 12, about surviving parental separation and divorce (Rees 2005, 2008). Ishmael Beah wrote about his time as a boy soldier in a story relevant to many asylum-seeking children and young people in the UK (Beah 2007).

Service user stories have a unique power and many should be prescribed reading on courses about partnership working.

Redefined professional roles

New support brokerage models represent 'a change in power relationships, using a citizenship model which defines people who use services as contributors and partners rather than as dependent recipients', and can be contrasted to the traditional 'professional gift' model of support, according to Carl Poll, an In Control service user advocate. The broker is a fundamentally different role from care manager and social worker before them, a slow process of redefining social work and social care roles in a difficult balancing act between protection, social control and empowerment (GSCC 2007). Safe and constructive role redefinition can be supported by social valorisation training, which concentrates on bringing out the personal strengths of service users, rather than a deficit model. Unless this is done, people using services will not become 'commissioners of their own care' (Integrated Care Network 2008), but rather will continue 'to be viewed as vulnerable people in need of care, instead of active valued citizens, in charge of our own lives' (Campbell 2008).

Service-user-led partnership working is matched in other fields, particularly technology, where 'clients demand technology blends that oblige providers to collaborate' (Mulholland *et al.* 2007).

The constraints on an empowerment model, and the dilemmas facing social care professionals, relate primarily to managing risk and resources (see also Chapter 1). For example, someone at risk of suicide or harming a child, or a vulnerable adult will need to be controlled first and supported later. During the course of an average working day, a social care worker, and indeed all front-line staff whatever their role, may have to be supportive, analytical, decisive, reflective and confrontational, depending on the situations they face.

Tensions between service users and professionals

Rhetoric about partnerships disintegrates if the basic level of service provided and received is poor. Take the central notion of a partnership between a social worker and a child looked after. The abiding principle since the 1948 Children Act has been one child, one social worker – for the duration of a child's time in care, which is five to six years on average. Very few local authorities meet this standard, and some children looked after can be faced with a change in social worker several times a year. 'The longest I had a social worker was three months, then from there I've had 14 different social workers. It's hard because you get to know and trust one and it leaves' (Morgan 2007).

A climate of partnership can be undermined by a sense that a statutory organisation is not providing the level of service it should be. For example, couples denied IVF treatment because they live in the wrong part of the country feel they are being denied the service they have been paying taxes for because of a postcode lottery (Infertility Network UK 2007). Fourteen councils are working with the LGA, IdEA, RDAs and the National Foundation for Educational Research and Research in Practice, to look at the outcomes of integrated children's services, after initial work confirmed a wide variation in services. An equal suspicion and mistrust arises when the criteria for NHS continuing care are applied differentially by geography, and differently by clinicians, so that one person will be looked after free of charge if the NHS takes responsibility, and one will pay fees to a local authority if the NHS doesn't and if the care is deemed social care provided by a local authority and as a result chargeable.

Variations in performance between and within schools in England is significantly above OECD averages. Variations within schools are between five and fourteen times greater than between school variance, with a study in Dallas showing that the performance gap between students assigned three effective teachers in a row, and those assigned three ineffective teachers, was as much as 49 per cent (Sanders and Rivers 1996). The same span of competence applies to a greater or lesser degree in every profession, the link to partnership working being that an effective professional is likely to achieve a stronger partnership with some one using a service, as they will get more done for the person they work with or for.

Perceptions that the service they have received is poor or unfair leads many service users to complain formally to their care providers.

> With no schooling from the age of 13, Amaryllis Mogaji, now 21, is angry at her lost opportunities and would like to sue her local authority, if only to make them pay for college classes. She left care at 18 but effectively left many years earlier. Whilst she accepts she was not easy to 'look after', she feels she is now left with nothing and that her period in care should be revived now and re-instituted for two more years to get her back on track in the crucial young adult years.
>
> (*Times Educational Supplement*, 17 March 2006)

Complaints procedures are an important protection for service users, and they should feature a strong independent element if initial problem-solving fails.

After-care partnerships

After an incident when a friend of mine woke up to find burglars in her bedroom making off with her jewellery, the local police visited her twice to make sure she was OK. For her, this mattered as much as finding the criminals. The thought of the police providing after-care for victims changed her view of the police. As the poet W. B. Yeats said, 'death is for the relatives', and how relatives are treated by agencies is crucial, including after mistakes or tragedies when a service user dies, through suicide or being murdered in circumstances where professionals risk being accused of negligence. Continuing to communicate openly with a family is an important sign of caring and good governance. Organisations should take a long-term interest and responsibility for staying in touch with families years after serious events. Memories of tragedies rarely fade, and family members can continue to have questions to ask and resolve years later, as do professionals.

Partnerships with carers

The vast majority of carers are ordinary family members, so their partnership with each other is the largest single partnership for state agencies to support. Helping family members to improve their own communication, including the resolution of any long-standing conflicts, can ensure the highest possible number of vulnerable people continue to be looked after and supported by family and/or friends. Linking back to the last section, parents of course are carers of their own children, and professionals can engage them as equals, rather than leave them to speculate about the potential damage from a social care intervention. Local Surestart programmes are committed to the involvement of parents, 'both as users and in the governance of the programmes', through parents being on all local Surestart Partnership Boards (Wigfall *et al.* 2007). This high level of parental involvement can be carried from Surestart programmes to their successor programmes in local children's centres – Surestart programmes are scheduled to be 'mainstreamed' into local children's centres by 2010. As ' organisations with a memory', partnerships have to ensure that the learning from a predecessor agency is carried forward into the new agency and applied to service provision and development.

Formal caring is normally defined in terms of time spent, or the volume and complexity of physical tasks carried out. Emotional support is as important, though largely immeasurable. The higher profile service users and their carers have today compared with 20 years ago means that just as those in need of services, especially private payers, can define what help they want, so family carers are entitled to an assessment of their own needs when their caring role is substantial in time, effort and worry – though Carers UK suggested that only one third of carers entitled to this actually receive an assessment of their needs (Carers UK 2005).

Carers' support groups play a crucial role in directly supporting carers, in advocating for individual carers who need help, and in lobbying on carer's issues. Like all such support groups, they need close working partnerships with a range of influential people and organisations in order to maximise their effectivness.

Carers can be as young as seven or over 90. Young carers can be looking after one or both parents, without anyone realising it, despite a higher contemporary profile for young carers. Many carers in their nineties continue to look after their children with disabilities, who themselves may be in their seventies. Those carers generally want a partnership with the state which clearly sets out what will happen to their child or children when they die. Many local authorities are unable to guarantee a specific caring option or resources in advance, which causes older carers considerable anxiety.

Foster carers, or adopters or special guardians for children in care, need a combination of support, including mentoring and round-the-clock access to support workers, specialist advice, and adequate funding, as 'living and working with children who have lived through maltreatment presents carers and workers with profound puzzles. We need to be able to make sense of the chaos the children bring into our lives' (Cairns 2002). Most foster carers and adoptive parents today are therapeutic parents. Fostering support agencies can support foster carers in many different ways, like Southwark Council's support for foster carers enhancing their own educational ability so that they in turn can support the children and young people they look after in

Suffolk Family Carers – going from strength to strength

Suffolk Family Carers now employs 64 staff, double the number five years ago. They have also diversified, to provide an increasing number of services, including a mental health project, a young carers support group, a black and ethnic minority support group, as well as teams in hospitals and a well-used helpline and website. Their chief executive, Jacqui Martin, networks hard and is a key member of a number of local statutory partnerships (see 'Statutory partnerships' below). They have found carers increasingly hard pressed for four reasons:

- care needs are becoming more complex, with the rise in long-term conditions a key factor
- earlier discharges from hospital and shorter periods in respite care add to the carer's burden
- they sense less flexibility in the workplace than there used to be, with workers who are also carers less able to take time off through pressure of work
- carers are increasingly having to pay more with state benefits not keeping pace with costs.

They also feel these changes in the nature of the caring task and the cared-for person have family consequences which are not generally understood. For example, professionals assume that end-of-life care for terminally ill patients should be at home, as most people would prefer to die at home rather than in care. However, this can be unbearably painful for relatives, including young children if they are in the house at the time. Partnership working today needs to take a more holistic family-centric view, not just to pursue the 'personalisation' agenda for the cared for person at any cost.

These pressures jeopardise the reciprocity and negotiation at the heart of family caring, an interdependence and two-way balancing act characterised by Bretheny and Stephens as 'resisting the decline and disengagement often associated with dependence ... an inter-dependence involving families negotiating roles and responsibilities actively as family members age' (Bretheny and Stephens 2007).

improving their educational performance in ways such as 'paired reading', as well as building up their resilience.

Such family placement partnerships can include continuous and simultaneous partnerships between the following:

- birth parents and social worker(s)
- birth mothers (tummy mummies) and their children
- birth fathers and their children
- birth grandparents and other relatives and the children
- birth children with each other
- adoptive parents and their adopted child/children
- adoptive parents and their own child/children
- adoptive parents and their social worker(s)
- adoptive parents and birth parents.

Foster care placements for mothers and babies are the most successful reunification placement for young mothers with major social problems and their babies (unpublished research by Elaine Farmer, University of Bristol), whereas overall 47 per cent of children who go home are back in care within one year.

Many structural issues for carers remain unresolved, such as lower payments or fees for carers of adults than for carers of children, and the variation in support from statutory agencies, ranging from 24-hour, round-the-clock support for some carers, to minimal or non-existent support for others. The concept of 'carer' itself, 'translates poorly into minority languages, so that even if needs are universal, solutions are different' (Afiya Trust 2008).

Communication breakdown is often at the heart of problems facing carers. When I worked with groups of carers, including foster carers and family carers, the meetings frequently started out with concerns about a lack of resources, but usually ended up complaining about poor communication with professional staff: complaints about not being informed, of being taken for granted, and of hostile or indifferent attitudes. By contrast, professional staff with good communication skills were usually able to solve most problems, leaving carers feeling supported and empowered. As Anne Parker, the former Director of Social Services in Berkshire, said after meeting a group of carers, 'I was really worried about meeting all of you tonight because I was afraid you would ask for services I can't provide because of my budget. I'd come with figures explaining my shortage of resources. But I am ashamed by how little you have asked for – really just a bit more recognition and understanding' (private conversation).

Statutory partnerships

Statutory partnerships are usually established many years after concerns start to be expressed about a cross-cutting social problem. The sequence starts with escalating local concerns, often media-fuelled, in many parts of the country, leading to a high profile review being set up by the government of the day. Following that, a new national strategy is written, consulted upon and launched, with the statutory partnership being the way it is finally implemented locally. That whole process can take between two and five years.

Education improvement partnerships; road safety partnerships; crime and disorder reduction partnerships; strategic health partnerships; local strategic partnerships; drug and alcohol action teams; local safeguarding children's boards: these are some of the plethora of partnerships in place across England, set up in broadly the same way irrespective of place. Scotland, Wales and Northern Ireland, whilst emphasising they are different, adopt similar approaches as cross-cutting issues don't stop at the border. The Strategic Partnerships in Manchester and Edinburgh use nearly identical frameworks and include the equivalent partner agencies, invariably from the public, private and third sectors.

The number of such strategies and partnerships is rising inexorably and exponentially, including the most recent strategy at the time of writing, to combat childhood obesity (Department of Health 2008), which will be another major and long-running cross-sector partnership. Whilst it seems inefficient that each part of the UK, over 200 local areas in all, develops its own strategy for everything, when each has far more similarities than differences, it is the process of local partners working together to create, produce, own and implement a local strategy that is irreplaceable. Whilst some organisations collaborate well across geographical boundaries, such as the London Safeguarding Children Board, to which all 33 London boroughs are signed up, most local leaders resent being told another part of the country does something better than they do, and that learning from elsewhere will translate easily to their situation. As L. P. Hartley (1953) wrote, 'the past is a foreign country; they do things differently there' and this is true of partnership development. Each area has to develop its own customized version of partnership working.

Government policy is to consolidate many statutory partnerships into a single framework, through Local Area Agreements and Multi-Area Agreements, but sensible rationalisation is still lacking.

Many partnerships end up simply feeding the information-seeking-and-spewing beast, and the central activity becomes bureaucratic – writing and reviewing business plans, work programmes, action plans and writing funding bids. The means can easily become the end. Other traits to avoid include agency representatives attending meetings merely to protect their own organisation or sector, frequently using wrecking tactics to delay a measure, and 'boosterism', in which individual agencies over-state their own contribution, primarily as self-justification (Perri 6 and Leat 1997).

Statutory or strategic partnerships need to guard against 'the document production industry' and 'find a way to get into real implementation and change' … 'turning process into output and outcomes' (Monmouthshire County Council 2007). Inspired by the Biblical proverb, 'locusts have no king, yet they advance together in ranks', it identified the following constraints on partnership working:

- complex and overwhelming partnership structures
- a focus on process rather than outcomes
- power imbalances
- partnership burnout
- lack of community and neighbourhood engagement
- an implementation gap.

The locust metaphor was used to place an emphasis on self-organising networks, aimed at building ' collaborative gain'. Monmouthshire County Council itself brought in a performance management system based on the delivery of citizen and community outcomes, rather than partnership processes.

Despite the risks and dangers, many Partnership Boards have made a contribution to community health and well being that would not have otherwise been achieved. A multi-agency coalition of agencies is tackling joblessness in Greater Manchester. Sheffield Safeguarding Children's Board Licensing Project has developed a licensing partnership with pubs and clubs, providing vetting checks to ensure people running premises are fit to do so – the Licensing Act 2003 requires that licensees impose safeguarding measures wherever they are needed. A related partnership project is 'Wasted', a responsible-drinking programme between a community organisation, Cragrats, based in Holmfirth, West Yorkshire, and Diageo, the world's leading alcoholic drinks business. The main programme is a tour of hundreds of schools, reaching thousands of pupils with messages and information about responsible drinking. Afterwards, young people reported the following outcomes (Cragrats 2007):

- 95 per cent of participants said the programme made them think about the effects of alcohol abuse
- 91 per cent learned more about how alcohol misuse can damage your health
- 88 per cent felt they could deal better in a situation where someone pressured them to drink alcohol.

Partnership working with shopkeepers to prevent sales of alcohol to young teenagers is another low-key yet significant everyday prevention measure.

The glue in statutory partnerships

Margaret Thatcher famously said of the Russian leader at the time, Mikhail Gorbachev, 'I think we can do business together'. The importance of interpersonal relationships between leaders of organisational power blocs within statutory partnerships should not be underestimated. Indeed, many partnerships stand or fall on the strength of personal relationships within or across organisations. The ability to compromise and see what is in front of you from the point of view of someone else is crucial in statutory partnerships. The 15 members of the Colchester 2020 strategic partnership are asked to leave their professional hats at the door when they meet as a body. Equally, at the team level, whilst alliances and friendship subgroups are inevitable, these have to be kept in check if a team is to function well. Mintzberg drew attention to the importance of the communication process at all levels of organisations and between organisations, if collaboration is to be genuine (Mintzberg *et al.* 1996).

Joint working between professional groups

Why it matters so much

One major factor in successful partnerships is the degree of ease felt by professional groups who work alongside each other on a daily basis. As Peck and Crawford found, in a study of the first care trusts in England:

> it is apparent that health and local government organisations and staff approach new partnership arrangements with well-established perceptions – both positive and negative – of each other. These perceptions, and in particular the differences, are often expressed in terms of culture. Further, it is clear culture plays a major roles in the success or failure of merged organisations.
>
> (Peck and Crawford 2004)

Dismantling defensive structural barriers and respecting separate cultures en route to formulating a shared narrative requires an understanding of why those barriers are functional for the people behind them. The reasons for barriers include: specific funding streams, professional allegiances, uncertainty about role and accountability, loss of autonomy and lack of consensus about purpose (Edwards 2007). Barriers make sense to those erecting them, even if they make no sense to anyone watching. The difficulty with some barriers between organisations is that they were put up by a past regime in a forgotten era, and even though the professionals behind the barriers would like to jump over them, they find themselves unable to, being now hemmed in by restrictive practices, policies and procedures.

Co-locating joint services can break down this type of barrier, through relationships. Traditional professional adversaries, opthalmologists and optometrists, describe how this shift took place within the Fife Interdisciplinary Low Vision Service (FILVS), including an eye surgeon becoming much more aware of the patient, not just their eyes, through working together over a period of time with a sensory impairment support worker (*The Guardian*, 23 April 2008). Similarly, identifying with a new joint team, rather than predecessor teams, can be unifying, as Douglas and Philpot found in a family partnership team in Kensington and Chelsea, where 'education professionals

Police officers and social workers talking about each other

'I write down everything they [social workers] say. I've found them to be liars' – a woman police officer in a joint police/children's social services child protection team.

'80 per cent are very good, but 20 per cent only worry about themselves and create hassles. This 20 per cent have what I call "attitude problems" ... they're always running to their line managers' – another police officer in the team.

'If they're interviewing a child and they think the child might not be telling the truth [about an allegation of abuse], it's very difficult for them because all their training tells them to approach interviewing in a very confrontational way, yet we know that this is not very helpful for the child' – a social worker in the team.

'As as I'm concerned, I'm servicing the police. I'm trying to get a child to tell me what happened, so there's a weight of evidence for my police colleagues to go and confront a guy with' – another social worker in the team.

Despite this, traditional barriers between professions are being broken down, partly due to a growing culture of support for joint working. In 2008, one of the most senior police officers in Northern Ireland, Assistant Chief Constable Peter Sheridan, left to become Chief Executive of Co-operation Ireland, a cross-border charity promoting better relations between all-Irish communities and people north and south of the border. At the same time, Adrian McAllister, acting Deputy Chief Constable of Lancashire police, became the first Chief Executive of the Independent Safeguarding Authority for England. Senior police officers rarely used to move between sectors, but an increasing number of senior professionals, more comfortable in the inter-agency world than their predecessors, are now doing do.

(All quotes Garrett 2003)

saw the team as an education resource, health professionals saw it as a health resource and social workers as a social services resource. Everyone thought the service belonged to them' (Douglas and Philpot 1998).

A survey (Barbour *et al.* 2003) of 500 practitioners working in community mental health services found that:

- GPs and adult psychiatrists found it most difficult to coordinate their work and were most likely to experience problems in respect of confidentiality
- child care social workers were most likely to identify problems of co-ordination with psychiatrists
- community care support workers, community psychiatric nurses, approved social workers and community mental health centre staff reported fewer problems of co-ordination.

Studies such as this show that higher status professionals often have the most difficulty in working together, preferring the company of each other rather than professionals they think are in a less serious, or a less academic or a less important profession. Whilst this is nothing short of professional snobbery, it is another barrier with a purpose – this time to maintain status differentials.

Whilst Olive Stevenson identified tensions between police and social workers as particularly sensitive, no professional group wants its status and expertise to be diluted, because so much of the identity of individual professionals is located in the values and identity of the profession they trained in and have come to love (Stevenson 1994). Sims, Fineman and Gabriel suggest that 'professionalism is a systematic body of knowledge with monopoly powers over its applications' (Sims *et al.* 1993). Pollard, Miers and Gilchrist found that students on pre-qualifying courses are hostile to collaborative working in health and social care, because each profession views itself more positively than it does other professions (Pollard *et al.* 2004). Frost found 'familiar stereotypes of over-anxious health visitors and teachers facing impassive social workers' (Frost 2005). Most professions have their own initiation rites, private language and set of arcane practices into which new entrants are swiftly socialised, even if they arrive wanting to change the world. Indeed, without a compellingly articulated partnership vision, legacy cultures may survive intact inside new partnership teams or organisations.

Reducing resistance to partnership working

Working in small groups, with a practice focus, helps to reduce negative stereotyping between professional groups, and in one major study which contrasted uni-professional and inter-professional learning, 'most student groups from practice based initiatives were cohesive irrespective of the nature of professional membership. Few reported negative stereotyping' (Miller *et al.* 2006).

Joint training programmes are important as training is 'one of the few processes which might successfully operate in the 'spaces between organisations' (Howarth and Glennie 1999).

Relationship development between professional groups inside multi-disciplinary teams benefits from a structured approach to breaking down barriers. One community mental health team for older people took the following steps (Miller and Wallman-Durrant 2001):

- defined the key-worker role as a generic role, opening it up to all professional disciplines represented in the team, thus recognising the value of each
- took time out for team development on a regular basis, including away-days and team meetings
- conducted value clarification exercises, affirming the values team members shared
- achieved clarity about role and task differentiation
- trained the team in service developments like person-centred planning in dementia care.

The crucial role of supervision

Tony Morrison found that 'supervision is crucial for negotiating around inter-professional difference' and that 'it is crucial that interdisciplinary leaders handle difference well'. Giving regular reflective supervision to members of professional groups like health visitors who are used to receiving much less, because of the wider span of control of primary health care managers, can help those staff feel more at home in a joint team (Tony Morrison, independent child welfare trainer and consultant 2007).

The supervision relationship is a partnership.

The partnership should:	and should not:
• be a continuous process	• be a one off event
• encourage and involve you	• undermine you
• recognise your good performance and personal achievements	• avoid challenge where this is needed
• help you to be clear about your roles and responsibilities	• confuse you
• be structured and focused	• include 'small talk and cosy chat'
• identify the resources you need to do the job	• make unfair demands
• be planned and private	• be rushed or interrupted
• be a two way process	• be one-sided
• focus on your individual needs	• focus on the supervisor's needs
• be motivating	• feel negative or demoralizing
• address professional development	• ignore the right and need for development
• be confidential, subject to the safety of people or staff	• break confidentiality
• deal with situations sensitively and clearly	• ignore or fail to support you

'The supervisor–worker relationship is the key encounter where the influence of organisational authority and professional identity collide and connect' (Middleman and Rhodes 1980).

Inter-professional joint development work

Designing a new integrated model of care can itself be the focus of a joint training programme and can lead to a stronger professional model. For example, a dementia care model can include the latest drug treatment where applicable, support for carers, person centred planning with people using services, and potentially their carer(s) as well, occupational therapy, and a specialist architect to ensure the home environment is suitably designed and adapted. An integrated model for assessment and care planning can still be supplemented by guidance for individual professional staff in their own professional discipline.

Without developmental work, and a deliberate change in working practices towards more inclusive working between professional groups, real or perceived power imbalances will inevitably continue, and lead to the resentment expressed by this health visitor:

> 'In one of my cases, a baby was removed. I'd been working on this case for eighteen months, we were working quite closely I thought. But all of a sudden the child was removed and it was a fortnight before somebody got on the phone to me and said, "oh, by the way, we've removed the child'. I thought, am I part of this, or what?'
>
> (Harlow and Shardlow 2006)

At the Level 2 Youth Centre in Felixstowe, Suffolk, a health visitor mingles freely with young people, subtly pairing off with one for an impromptu counselling session in a sideroom about sexual health or pregnancy fears. If young people won't go to a clinic, the clinic has to go to young people. This is one of thousands of projects and mainstream services where inter-professional working is of a high standard. Many professionals enjoy working with someone from another discipline, and see it as adding value to what they do. In Cafcass, many judges and Cafcass practitioners work together at court in private law cases, providing a dispute resolution service to separated parents who cannot agree on the arrangements for care of their children. The judiciary and Cafcass have separate independent roles prescribed by statute, yet can work together constructively, with success rates for safe agreements between parents standing at between 60 per cent and 70 per cent throughout England and Wales. In a similar way, the signatures of an approved social worker (ASW) and an adult psychiatrist are required before a vulnerable adult can be compulsorily admitted to a psychiatric unit under s3 of the Mental Health Act 1983. The two professionals will agree on some cases and disagree on others, but they manage to sit alongside each other in community mental health teams up and down the country as colleagues – most of the time anyway.

It is not just the professional groups in constant contact with each other, like social workers, health visitors, GPs, community nurses and teachers, who need to work together. Architects play a crucial role in designing good care environments, particularly in dementia care homes to ensure resident satisfaction and safety. This might involve creating internal and external walkways which allow residents to wander in any direction without meeting barriers but crucially, without being able to wander out of the home – in a figure of eight, for example – or creating tramlines for wheelchairs down cobbled paths and streets. Firefighters run courses in fire stations to teach teenagers problem-solving skills as well as firefighting skills, which would have been unheard of partnership working a decade ago. In a partnership between Berwick Surestart and the Northumberland Fire and Rescue Service, Surestart outreach staff including a health visitor, midwives and a play worker, operate out of the retained fire station in Wooler, central Northumberland. Firefighters carry out home safety assessments and are involved in other joint programmes. As a positive spin-off, setting up child care services for some firefighters led to success in recruiting women firefighters.

At the heart of good inter-professional working is an understanding of the pressures on one another. Communication between the police and social workers over child protection cases improved when formal structured joint investigations and joint child protection teams were established in the 1980s. According to Roger Graef, the fly-on-the-wall documentary film maker and criminologist, police officers are under great pressure to match the fictional account of what they do, recreated several times each day on TV in police dramas which emphasise successful detection. Graef claims police officers real working lives are not aligned with the public narrative about what they do. They are, he claims, living in a script in which they're the hero, whereas in reality they are poor at crime detection but good at problem-solving, spending most of their time unglamorously on the street or in people's homes dealing with people who are drunk, who have mental health problems or who demonstrate anti-social behaviour (Graef 1982). Inter-professional working requires professionals to understand what each other's daily jobs are really like, without stereotyping. This implies mature co-existence rather than going native or shutting a profession out. As Parker found, 'cultural management in the sense of creating an enduring set of shared beliefs is impossible' (Parker 2000). Mature co-existence is the natural state.

Inter-professional standards and codes of practice can support new partnership values, such as the General Social Care Council's 'Statement of Inter-professional Values Underpinning Work with Children and Young People' (GSCC 2007), and The English National Board for Nursing and CCETSW's joint strategy for shared learning which supported integrated working practices (ENB and CCETSW 1992).

Partnerships and organisations

Partnerships across organisations

Partnership working requirements on statutory organisations are multiplying relentlessly, for the right reasons but often without an implementation plan, which usually means the approach is hit or miss. In new public service agreements from April 2008, Primary Care Trusts are expected to pool budgets with local authorities to improve adolescent health outcomes, and Youth Offending Teams are expected to pool 10 per cent of their budget with local support services for young person's initiatives. In England, government departments have acquired joint responsibility for cross-cutting issues and services – the Department of Children, Schools and Families (DCSF) and the Department for Culture, Media and Sport (DCMS) for play, and DCSF and the Ministry of Justice (MOJ) for youth justice. A new breed of civil servants with partnership working responsibilities written into their job briefs is springing up in central government – a decade after they started in earnest in local agencies. At the time of writing, 29 out of the 30 Public Service Agreements for central government were cross-departmental.

A compelling reason to improve partnership working is the likelihood all politicians and professionals will have to cope with it at some point during their career, and probably sooner rather than later. At the time of writing, 30 out of 32 Scottish councils are coalitions of local political parties – and all possible permutations at that – necessitating collaborative working between traditional opponents. Glasgow and Edinburgh councils, 'Glasburgh', once old enemies, have jointly appointed an 'inter-city tsar' to run a twin cities project focusing on how best to collaborate and not compete.

Working in partnership is a contradiction in terms for some professionals, who prize independence above every other value. Judges for example are not just independent from other organisations and government, they are independent from each other, which often makes joint working with the judiciary, vital in some programmes, a conceptual impossibility.

Some academics do not engage enough with other academics working on similar issues across schools, e.g. a law school and a psychology school, not necessarily through malice, but through unfamiliarity with the principles and advantages of partnership working.

Partnerships within organisations

Partnership working involves building horizontal bridges across organisations and networks (Casto 1994). Yet internal partnership working is equally important. A strong and cohesive internal partnership culture can produce a higher level of performance than a fragmented and unhappy one. 'The reality is that internal relationships are often worse than external relationships. Internal relationships can be treated with contempt with functions trying

Bromley Priory School

As part of the remodelling process at Bromley Priory School in Orpington, Kent, support staff were given the opportunity to achieve Level 1 and 2 Vocational Qualifications. Some are working towards Level 3. The school's performance at KS3 and GCSE has improved substantially. The significant aspect of the change is the fact that teachers were able to focus much more on teaching and learning.

Source: Department for Children, Schools and Families 2008

to gain advantage over each other. Good interdepartmental relationships perform better in terms of meeting customer needs, accommodating special customer requests and introducing new services and products' (Wilding 2006). Support roles like teaching assistants, legal assistants and special constables are now becoming fully fledged professional roles in themselves, and the partnership between fully qualified and less qualified professionals needs to be well-supported within organisations, as it can bring benefits to service users (see 'Bromley Priory School' box above).

Partnerships between managers and front-line staff

I recently talked to a retiring official from the electricity industry, a manager from Thames Water, a group of telecoms technicians and a BBC executive. All complained wryly and occasionally bitterly about low morale in their organisations caused by, in the case of the electricity and water industries, privatisation and subsequently take-overs by American and Australian companies respectively, and in the case of the BBC, by the domineering approach of executives with no roots in the industry who distrusted professional broadcasters. Another friend who had worked for a multi-national all his life as a specialist engineer, was upset to have 'lost' his head office – he no longer knew where it was – and to have 'lost' his professional autonomy, in that before undertaking any repair work he now had to phone his new call centre to gain approval, from someone with far less experience than him. Some NHS clinicians refer to NHS management as 'the dark side'.

An effective partnership between managers and front-line staff is crucial. In 1985, the engineers on the NASA space programme knew there were countless risk areas within the design of the Challenger space shuttle. They were especially concerned about the O ring seals which they were worried would fail – they did, causing the death of seven astronauts. Engineers claimed managers ignored their advice because they did not want any delays in the programme. Just as practitioners can feel pulled in every direction, and be refused the discretion to interpret central directives that street-level bureaucrats need (Lipsky 1980), managers can experience regular 'brainfry' and be subjected, sometimes by taking on more than they can manage, to role confusion and overload. These conflicts, if they occur simultaneously, can lead to communication breakdowns or even the collapse of a service.

The strength of the psychological contract between staff and their employing organisation, for example between social care staff out and about on their own in the community, facing pressures and risks, and their 'motherships', can make the difference between a contented and discontented professional. All too often, staff are employed for their strengths and managed for their weaknesses. Strengths-based approaches to management and partnership working can motivate staff more, especially in a time of rapid change and constraints on professional discretion with more emphasis on consistency and uniformity of approach. This can lead to the disillusionment expressed by Napier:

> So why have I become so deeply ashamed of my job and of my employer that I am considering leaving a field of work that I have enjoyed for so long? If Britain cannot provide for the most vulnerable people, and we condone the constant shifting of the goalposts, such as the definition of the 'vulnerable', then we should all be deeply ashamed. I know I am. And if I look around at all the wealth in the UK and can still look someone straight in the eye and tell them that their care package is to be cut due to lack of funds, then I have betrayed every single one of the principles and ideals that brought me into this job in the first place.
>
> (Napier 2007)

Partnerships between peers

Practitioner-led partnerships are one way of increasing ownership of social care by social care workers. The Early Communication Screening Tool devised in Barnsley by speech and language therapists Margaret Pratt and Nicola Wilson, led to new assessment forms being introduced, which with continued observation and discussion, helped health professionals to make earlier decisions about referral on to specialist agencies.

The inter-relationship between front-line practitioners, support staff such as administrators, managers and specialists is vital to get right, especially when lives are at stake. 'The fax had sat for an hour too long in someone's in tray', illustrates how getting the right piece of paper to the right person at the right time is often crucial in safeguarding service users, when sometimes an hour is the difference between life and serious injury or death. As much paper is handled by administrators as practitioners, so the need for constant and effective communication is central. Administrators are often taken for granted. As a result, they can too easily become de-motivated. Their role in successful partnership working is crucial.

Peer support is the main source of support for social care staff. Staff working under pressure need their team bases to be sanctuaries, even for snatched conversations over a quick coffee – this holds true for every job, every profession and every sector. Organisations need to understand the value of peer support and peer relationships, as a first step to finding practical ways of giving them status, recognition and encouragement.

Partnerships across countries and cultures

The complexity of the modern social care task is the main reason for new partnerships between professional groups and organisations, including responding to the challenges of providing high quality social care services to diverse communities. Exchanges between health specialists in Rochdale, Lancashire and Sahiwal in Pakistan helped to increase the understanding of health needs and cultural and family structures. Some Asian families find it hard to accept dementia in a family member, as if it is becomes widely known in their community, they fear it will adversely affect the marriage prospects of young women in the family. A greater understanding of the links between culture and behaviour is vital to providing public services to ethnic minority groups.

The Alzheimer's Society is part of a global twinning programme managed by Alzheimer's Disease International (ADI), the umbrella organisation of Alzheimer's associations around the world, including partnerships between Los Angeles and Mexico, and Pakistan and Western Australia, aimed at pooling knowledge (*Share*, the Alzheimer's Society newsletter, July 2007).

The *Working Visits to Ghana* programme is a partnership between young people from Gateshead, supported by Connexions Tyne and Wear, Gateshead Council, Madventurer, Deckham Community Association, Ultimate Youth and people from the village of Shia in the Volta Region in Ghana. The aim is to promote young people as positive change makers and as active global citizens. Some of the young people who went from Gateshead in 2001, returned to Ghana in 2006, to assess the impact they had made.

Rapid social change (see Chapter 2), particularly through globalisation, has brought with it an explosion of new organisations and opportunities for partnership working. Steve Grout is a social worker living in Valencia, Spain, who set up a service called Key Professionals, which offers an assessment and advisory service to UK social care agencies who need to work with a family member living in Spain. This gives the opportunity of a local kinship care assessment where a member of the child's extended family lives permanently in Spain, rather than social workers in the UK going out to Spain on a one-off visit to make an assessment that is best carried out over a period of weeks or months by the same social worker.

These examples show the increasing globalisation of partnerships, in the interests of UK service users.

References

Afiya Trust, 2008, *Beyond We Care: Putting Black Carers in the Picture*, London: National Black Carers and Carers Workers Network.

Barbour, R., Stanley, N., Penhale, B. and Holden, S., 2002, 'Assessing risk: professional perspectives on work involving mental health and child care services', *Journal of Inter-professional Care*, 16(4): 323–34.

Beah, I., 2007, *A Long Way Gone: Memoirs of a Boy Soldier*, London: Fourth Estate.

Begum, N., 2006, *Doing it for Themselves: Participation and Black and Ethnic Minority Service Users*, London: Social Care Institute for Excellence.

Bretheny, M. and Stephens, C., 2007, *Older Adults's Experience of Family Life, Linked Lives and Independent Living*, Wellington: New Zealand Families Commission.

Cafcass, 2007, *Golden Standards of Practice in Working with Muslim Young People*, London: Cafcass.

Cairns, K., 2002, *Attachment, Trauma and Resilience*, London: BAAF.

Campbell, J., 2008, 'Joined up thinking', *The Guardian*, Society supplement, 30 April.

Camus, A., 1942, *The Outsider*, Harmondsworth: Penguin.

Carers UK, 2005, *Facts about Carers*, London: Carers UK.

Casto, M., 1994, 'Inter-professional work in the USA: education and practice', in A. Leathard (ed.) *Going Inter-Professional*, London: Routledge.

Cooke, P., 2000, *Final Report on Disabled Children and Abuse*, Nottingham: Ann Craft Trust.

Cooke, P. and Standen, P.J., 2002, 'Abuse and disabled children: hidden needs?' *Child Abuse Review*, 11(1): 1–18.

Cragrats, 2007, *Alcohol Education Programme Reaches Over 100,000 Pupils* (available at: www.cragrats.uk.com/latest-news/latest-news-article.asp?id=59&category=csr).

Department for Children, Schools and Families, 2008, *Building Brighter Futures: Next Steps for the Children's Workforce*, London: Department for Children, Schools and Families.

Department of Health, 2008, *Healthy Weight, Healthy Lives: A Cross-Government Strategy for England*, London: Department of Health.

Douglas, A. and Philpot, T., 1998, *Caring and Coping*, London: Routledge.

Edwards, A., 2007, 'Partnership working and outcomes: a case of the hare and the tortoise', *Journal of Integrated Care*, 15(1): 24–6.

ENB and CCETSW, 1992, *Joint Strategy for Shared Learning*, London: UKCC.

Fathers Direct, 2005, *Working with Fathers*, London: Fathers Direct.

Frost, N., 2005, *Professionalism, Partnership and Joined-up Thinking: A Research Review of Front-Line Working with Children and Families*, Totnes: Research In Practice.

Garrett, P.M., 2003, *Re-making Social Work with Children and Families*, London: Routledge.

Graef, R., 1982, *Police*, BBC1 Television.

GSCC, 2007, *Statement Of Values Underpinning Inter-Professional Work With Children And Young People*, London: General Social Care Council.

Harlow, E. and Shardlow, S., 2006, 'Safeguarding children: challenges to the effective operation of core groups', *Child and Family Social Work*, 11(1): 65–72.

Hartley, L.P., 1953, *The Go-Between*, Harmondsworth: Penguin Classics.

Hitchen, S., 2007, 'The use of collaboration to produce more effective serious incident inquiry reports, Devon Partnership NHS Trust', *Journal of Integrated Care*, 15(6): 22–9.

Howarth, J. and Glennie, S., 1999, 'Inter-agency child protection training: gathering impressions', *Child Abuse Review*, 8: 200–6.

Infertility Network UK, 2007, Survey on behalf of the Department of Health, London: Department of Health, London.

Integrated Care Network, 2008, *Bringing the NHS and Local Government Together: A Practical Guide to Integrated Working*, 2008, London: Integrated Care Network (as part of the Care Services Improvement Partnership, Department of Health).

Jones, D.P.H., 2003, *Communicating with Vulnerable Children*, London: Gaskell.

Lipsky, M., 1980, *Street-level Bureaucracy*, New York: Russell Sage Foundation.

Middleman, R.R. and Rhodes, G.B., 1980, 'Teaching the practice of supervision', *Journal of Education for Social Work*, 16(3): 51–9.

Millen, J. and Wallman-Durrant, L., 2001, 'Multi-disciplinary partnership in a community mental health team', in V. White and J. Harris (eds) *Developing Good Practice in Community Care*, London: Jessica Kingsley.

Miller, C., Woolf, C. and Mackintosh, N., 2006, *Evaluation of Common Learning Pilots and Allied Health Professions First Wave Sites*, London: Department of Health.

Mintzberg, H., Jorgensen, J., Dougherty, D. and Wesley, F., 1996, 'Some surprising things about collaboration: knowing how people connect makes it work better', *Organisational Dynamics*, 25(1): 60–71.

Monmouthshire County Council, 2007, *Our Council*, Cwmbran: Monmouthshire County Council.

Morgan, R., 2007, *Looked After in England: How Children Living Away From Home Rate England's Care*, London: CSCI.

Mulholland, A., Thomas, C., Kurchina, P. with Woods, D., 2007, *Mashup Corporations*, New York: Evolved Technologist Press.

Napier, A., 2007, 'Deep sense of shame', *The Guardian*, Society supplement, 1 August.

Parker, M., 2000, *Organisational Culture and Identity*, London: Sage.

Pascal, B., 1669 [1995], *Pensées*, Harmondsworth: Penguin Classics.

Peck, E. and Crawford, A., 2004, *Culture in Partnerships: What do We Mean by it and what can We do about it?*, London: Integrated Care Network.

Peck, E. and Glasby, J., 2004, 'Care trusts: emerging themes and issues', in J. Glasby and E. Peck (eds), *Care Trusts: Partnership Working in Action*, Oxford: Radcliffe Medical Press.

Peers, J., 2003, *Asparagus Dreams*, London: Jessica Kingsley.

Perri 6 and Leat, D., 1997, 'Inventing the British voluntary sector by committee: From Wolfenden to Deakin', *Non-Profit Studies*, 1(2): 23–46.

Pollard, K., Miers, M. and Gilchrist, M., 2004, 'Collaborative learning for collaborative working?', *Health and Social Care in the Community*, 12(4): 346–58.

Reder, P. and Duncan, S., 2003, 'Understanding communication in child protection networks', *Child Abuse Review*, 12(2): 92–100.

Rees, L., 2005, *Help, Hope, Happiness*, Inverness: Aultbea Publishing Company.

Rees, L., 2008, *At Sixes and Sevens*, Inverness: Aultbea Publishing Company.

Ridge, M., 2008, *Breaking the Silence*, Dublin: Gill and Macmillan.

Sanders, W. and Rivers, J.C., 1996, *Cumulative and Residual Effects of Teachers on Future Student Academic Achievement*, Knoxville, TN: University of Tennessee Value-Added Research and Assessment Center.

Sims, D., Fineman, S. and Gabriel, Y., 1993, *Organising and Organisations: An Introduction*, London: Sage.

Stevenson, O., 1994, 'Child protection: where now for inter-professional work?', in A. Leatheard (ed.), *Going Inter-professional*, London: Routledge.

Timms, J., Bailey, S. and Thoburn, J., 2007, *Your Shout Too*, NSPCC Policy Practice Research Series, London: NSPCC.

Trivedi, P., 2002, 'Let the tiger roar', *Mental Health Today*, August: 30–3.

Waterhouse, R., 2000, *Lost in Care*, London: OPSI.

Watson, M., 2008, 'Social networking: an opportunity for health and social care?', *Journal of Integrated Care*, 16(1): 41–3.

Welbourne, P., 2002, 'Culture, children's rights and child protection', *Child Abuse Review*, 11(6): 345–58.

Wigfall, V., Boddy, J. and McQuail, S., 2007, 'Parental involvement: engagement with the development of services', in J. Schneider, M. Avis and P. Leighton (eds), *Supporting Children and Families*, London: Jessica Kingsley.

Wilding, R., 2006, 'Playing the tune of shared success', *Financial Times*, 10 November.

4 Who are the partners?

Part 2: Broader partnerships

Key messages

- Knowledge partnerships are crucial in a sector where knowledge is growing faster than educational institutions can teach it
- A wide range of partnerships can support social care staff in their work. Learning programmes need to make use of the options on offer in an increasingly global and 'knowledge-led' environment
- Teams around an issue or a service can make a massive difference
- One person can make a massive difference

Knowledge and learning partnerships

New technology and partnerships

Knowledge is the most valuable commodity 'owned' by successful organisations. 'Learning is the core capability for twentieth-century living', according to Professor Guy Claxton, Professor of the Learning Sciences at the University of Bristol Graduate School of Education. Knowledge partnerships are commonplace across sectors, like the triple helix partnerships between business, academia and government showcased in www.newcastlesciencecity. com.

Knowledge partnerships cross geographical boundaries, especially through their use of new technology. Britain's first virtual learning zone is the Kent/ Somerset virtual education zone, which will connect 11,000 students in 24 schools across two counties, providing computer and video links for students and teachers. Private-sector sponsors are contributing £250,000 a year. Knowledge transfer partnerships (KTPs) are growing in number, such as a DTI/EPSRC programme to encourage small to medium-sized British companies to collaborate with universities in innovative projects. Knowledge transfers from the University of East Anglia (UEA) include developing teamwork in a local NHS trust and helping a West Yorkshire Social Care service develop an in-house research strategy. The Bologna Process encourages joint degrees and qualifications frameworks between academic institutions across Europe, such as the partnership between the School of Nursing Midwifery and Social Care at Napier University Edinburgh and Hanze University in Groningen, the Netherlands, focusing on student mobility and exchange visits. All 22 local authorities in Wales are members of the Wales College of Research in Practice, which supports evidence-based practice.

M-learning (mobile phone applications) and e-learning (internet-based) are making some academic processes and buildings such as libraries virtually redundant. However, this in turn brings risks that information is becoming more random and disorganised, as learners just use the first page of a Google list to research and analyse a topic, rather than a list carefully assembled by experienced librarians.

Applying knowledge to social care practice

Doing a job well depends on what you know and how you apply it, especially in relation to evidence-based practice. June Thoburn, Emeritus Professor of Social Work at the University of East Anglia, said in relation to three child protection cases in which she had conducted inquiries: 'what matters is what they (professionals) should have known, not just what they should have done' (see for example Appendix 1 to the Inquiry Report on a Wakefield foster care case – Thoburn 2007).

Yet even today, many basic social care 'conditions' are still not being diagnosed properly, including mental health problems like depression, schizophrenia, stress and alcohol abuse faced by older people (UK Inquiry into Mental Health and Well-Being in Later Life 2007). On top of this, the main professional groups supporting older people with mental health problems disagree about which services need to be developed and lack a shared vision (Tucker *et al.* 2007).

Despite these limitations, social care as a profession knows a lot more about itself and its subject matter than it did 20 years ago. The knowledge base for areas as diverse as sexual abuse, complex disabilities and domestic violence have grown out of all recognition, from the time in 1973 when Maria Colwell was killed by her stepfather and the substance misuse problems in the Kemble/Colwell household were neither appreciated nor assessed. Pioneering work by a child psychologist in Gloucestershire, Robin Balbernie, has improved our understanding of 'the neurobiological consequences of early relationships' for children in need, and the irreversible physical damage that can be done to be development of a child's brain through a lack of attachment or abuse (Balbernie 2007). Thirty years ago, dyslexia was identified as a serious learning problem for children, whereas before it was recognised, children were seen as having conduct or behaviour problems. The same is true today in the recognition of dyscalculia, the equivalent learning difficulty in relation to number recognition. Recognition can bring understanding, reframing, re-classification and support for children and their parents. These are examples of knowledge breakthroughs in social care and related disciplines over the last few decades. Knowledge is easier to share and exchange in the public sector than in the private sector, where knowledge conveys commercial and competitive advantage and so is often kept secret.

The fact that the first three quotes in this section are from academics shows the central importance of academics to successful social care practice (also see later in this chapter). However, academics do not work in a vacuum. They need strong links with practice organisations through which to carry out research, particularly research into practice. A good example of inter-dependence in partnership working is the degree of collaboration between professional researchers and problem owners in social care agencies (Cairns *et al.* 2006). Collaboration between individual researchers and mainstream organisations can help to raise the profile of particular service user groups whose needs go unmet. *Towards joined-up lives* reported on the needs of disabled and deaf Londoners, in a research partnership between disabled people's research organisations and a mainstream research organisation. 'This partnership was brought together in recognition that organisations of disabled people often do not have the necessary capacity to deliver large-scale research projects and that mainstream research organisations often do not have a working understanding of social model methodology' (GLA 2006).

Knowledge partnerships recognise that each social care case is distinct and the knowledge needed for each particular case is likely to be specialist knowledge. In many ways, to paraphrase the novelist Evelyn Waugh who said 'there is no such thing as the man in the street' (Waugh 1953), there is no such thing as 'families, or 'mental health problems', or 'cultural types', there are just individuals with, in social care terms, their own unique 'DNA of difficulty' or 'uniquity'. Expert knowledge about each one is what social care can offer. Cases are also becoming more complex. A recent case I heard about involved an EU citizen who came to live and work in the UK, bringing with him a woman and her children he had 'bought' in Africa. He began sexually abusing one of the children, and it emerged he had been convicted of sexual offences in his European country of origin. The case will take months if not years to understand and unravel.

Knowledge about cases is often at a premium, such are the sheer number of specialist areas of knowledge needed to decipher a single case. Partnerships and communication through dialogue offer the best hope of approaching the 'truth' of a case. For example, in addressing issues of race and culture, a culture dialogic approach can help to understand such individuality. Melanie Henwood and Bob Hudson have highlighted some of the misplaced stereotypes about people who use services held by some social care professionals. They quote an interviewee who remarked, 'I have never yet met a parent whose child is going through transition who says "I want them to go to that day centre for the next 40 years and have the same key worker and the same friends doing the same thing every day". And I have not yet met an older person who says "I want to go and stagnate"' (Henwood and Hudson 2008).

Training partnerships

Partnership working brings with it considerable training needs, particularly for joint training between professional groups. New courses have started to address this need, such as the National Professional Qualification in Integrated Centre Leadership (NPQICL), the first programme to train children's centre leaders in multi-agency settings with integrated workforces like early years services. The move to an integrated qualifications framework for children's services staff means that some 4,000 qualifications will have to be sorted through by 2010. This will only work if the respective professional bodies and the vocational training sector play their part in the partnership.

Several local councils and universities have created partnership posts, such as Gloucestershire Social Services and the University of Gloucestershire, who host inter-agency seminars after work. In Berkshire, key research is summarised for staff on single laminated sheets. Social work programmes at master's and doctoral levels are establishing collaborative links and exchange schemes between academics, researchers and social work managers in countries with diverse needs and populations (McCrystal and Godfrey 2001).

A strong knowledge partnership draws in all staff. Without this, only a small percentage of staff take advantage of the training on offer in their agency. Frequently, the staff who need training most are also the most fearful or dismissive of it, so who is and who isn't taking up training opportunities needs monitoring. Like students who are learning, staff who are learning

Partnership for a purpose: forming a training collaborative to engage with provider organisations

A partnership between Tower Hamlets Council, the Learning and Skills Council (LSC) and the local Strategic Health Authority (SHA), allowed local home care organisations to meet the national care standards set out in the Care Standards Act 2000. Tower Hamlets used some of their National Training Strategy grant to pay replacement costs (payable to learners) to enable agency leaders to come to training events without losing pay. The SHA funded the assessor and administrative posts and the LSC funded a paperfree assessment system and met with every organisation to help them carry out a training needs analysis. The Profit from Learning initiative enabled Tower Hamlets as the lead agency to access free ESOL and Basic Skills training which enabled learners, especially in the local Bangladeshi community, to access the training and to be able to cope with the language. Most carers are non-traditional learners for whom English is a second language. The partnership shows what different partners may be willing to contribute to a project if they are constructively and positively engaged.

need time set aside to read and study. Some agencies grant staff a set number of days reading and reflection time, whatever the pressures, arguing that without that, practice will not improve.

Learning programmes are also being extended to service users, such as the Learning Opportunities Action Forum in Oldham, which supports people with mental health problems to access and participate in adult education.

Students and partnership working

The value of partnerships with higher educational institutions (HEIs) is shown by the many partnerships between HEIs and industry, particularly in product development. These have helped to develop state-of-the-art technology in engineering, pharmaceuticals and communications technology, to name just a few (Lisenburgh and Harding 2000). As social care seeks to develop stronger evidence bases, links with HEIs become more important, particularly with individual course leaders in the key areas for future practice requirements. Employer/university partnerships are often based on *learning agreements* signed by the employer, the employee, the assessor, and the university tutor, so that four people are 'signed up' to the success of an individual learning programme.

Education and training providers are increasingly willing to go into partnership with organisations to develop customised programmes such as e-learning packages. In addition to this, many HEIs offer modules in partnership working which count as credits towards a particular qualification, from NVQ up to master's level, including the University of East Anglia's School of Inter-professional Studies and the NHS University's School of Inter-professional practice. Learning is often applied to partnership working in a student or learner's own area of practice. Learning outcomes are usually mapped against the knowledge and skills framework competencies. For example, the learning outcomes from the 'Developing Partnership Working' master's module at the University of Teeside are:

- synthesise and integrate theories of partnership working and inter-disciplinary leadership
- demonstrate skills of creative and flexible thinking to be innovative in the development of integrated ways of working
- Analyse critically the complexities of partnership and integrated working in the context of the modernisation agenda
- evaluate critically the effectiveness of partnership and interdisciplinary working in the student's area of work
- critically evaluate and manage ethical issues related to collaborative practice, demonstrating emotional intelligence
- make a clear and concise presentation to peers.

Many social care agencies have a formal partnership with one or more academic providers, to provide short courses, to deliver post-qualifying training, or to second staff on to qualifying training at a higher education institution. Agencies may provide practice learning placements for students, so knowledge partnerships can be two-way, although it is still hard for many students to find a good practice placement, the more so since degree students on social work degree courses must do a minimum of 200 days of practice learning, up from 120 days for the previous Diploma in Social Work. Some agencies support students superbly. The Centre for the Development of Social Care, a partnership between Luton Council and the University of Bedfordshire, provides up to 8 students with a base for their second or final year of study, with use of computers, phones and interview rooms (*Community Care* 2006).

Research in partnership working has been usefully summarised by the Social Care Institute of Excellence (SCIE, 2006). They found the absence of a 'partnership curriculum', and that partnership working is 'under-theorised' with an absence of core texts, a lack of an empirical base, along with a sense of partnership working always being 'work in progress'. However, they also noted positive examples of good inter-professional learning, such as:

- dual qualifying programmes for joint practitioners or 'hybrid' workers, like the joint social work and nursing degree in learning disabilities at South Bank University
- a Service User and Carer group involved in the development of the social work degree at Dundee University, with formal representation in the programme structure
- the User and Carer Involvement Project at Anglia Ruskin University.

Courses such as the University of Birmingham's Health and Social Care Management Centre's (HSMC) Health and Social Care Partnerships Programme – the first of its kind in the country – also broke new ground.

Knowledge as the basis for improvement partnerships

Knowledge partnerships can be used to help improve performance. Kent and Swindon councils formed a partnership to use the expertise in social care services in Kent to raise standards in Swindon, which had received a series of poor inspection and audit reports. Similarly, every special school is to have a School Improvement Partner (SIP), who is to provide the school with support and challenge, mentored through the National College for School Leadership (NCSL). International knowledge exchanges are also developing. International Partnerships is a small UK charity helping China to develop its first foster schemes for orphaned children.

A similar knowledge partnership can work between an organisation and its regulator. Inspectors have the power to bring an entire organisation to a halt. The power of a small team of inspectors to induce paranoia in a regulated service, be it a day care service, a school, a care home or an entire service, is out of all proportion to the perceived impact inspectors feel they have. A 93-year-old woman I know went into respite care in a top rated private care home, only to be woken up at 7 a.m. the next morning for no apparent reason, being offered bread and butter and orange juice for breakfast, neither of which she likes, and not being given a bath throughout the first week because somehow 'she missed her turn'. Inspectors can only ever see a snapshot of what care is like, not what happens every day. Nor is it easy, despite a greater climate of openness, for service users or residents to express their views to outsiders for fear of repercussions, however much reassurance and promise of anonymity is granted.

Inspectors do bring about major changes in services, which is the underlying intention of a good regulator. There is little doubt that Ofsted has directly raised standards in schools over the last 20 years through its work. In 2003, several London boroughs were on 'special measures' for poor social services. By 2007, none were in this category. Of course improvement and recovery plans are developed and implemented by inspected services, not by regulators. But the presence of an inspection regime nearly always leads to that improvement or recovery plan being given top priority by the inspected services. Despite its inherent limitations, inspection and regulation is a crucial check and balance on the safety and quality of services to vulnerable people. Inspectors are in a concealed yet important partnership with people who use

---

The East London Consortium

The Consortium consists of four state schools and two independent schools for girls, with the City of London School for Girls taking the lead role. The schools learn from each other and work in partnership to help raise standards in education and 'narrow the gap' between the educationally advantaged and disadvantaged. Programmes include the Urban Scholars Intervention Programme (USIP), a Saturday school for up to 60 gifted and talented state school students, and 'Changing Lives', a project to raise aspirations and promote self-esteem in young women, run in partnership with the Women's Library and the London Metropolitan University. This involves students investigating the history of their own schools, collecting oral testimonies from former pupils and producing a documentary film on the history of campaigns led by inspirational women, from the nineteenth century social reformer, Josephine Black, to today's Southall Black Sisters, who campaign against domestic violence. Conferences and events play a big part in developing shared values through the consortium.

The Consortium is one of a number of innovative social and educational programmes in East London, following a long tradition of legendary centres for improvement and innovation like Toynbee Hall.

services, and increasingly they see the need to work collaboratively with those they inspect, to promote tailored improvement strategies.

An equally supportive approach underpins the work of improvement partnering in schools, including the Independent State School Partnership (ISSP), or Building Bridges, which started in 1997. This initiative, supported by the Children's University Programme, and now well developed in many areas, enables private and public schools to work together to share expertise, particularly to apply learning from the private schools sector to children and young people in less advantaged schools (see 'The East London Consortium' box above).

Partnerships with volunteers

Partnership working between the state and the third sector is sometimes set out in a series of strategic partnership agreements or 'compacts' – another keyword in the partnership working lexicon – which propose the involvement of the voluntary and community sector (VCS) in all new partnership structures (see 'Statutory partnerships' in Chapter 3).

A good example of a 'compact in action' is when Surrey County Council sold a closed school building to the Guildford-based charity, Disability Challengers, for less than market value because of the value the charity would add through building a £3 million play centre providing a range of leisure and play opportunities to 1,000 of the county's 4,000 children with disabilities. 50 per cent of costs were met by Surrey County Council, with the charity raising the rest through fund-raising.

Play and youth provision is just one of countless statutory services which would collapse overnight without the 2 to 3 million volunteers who keep local centres and services going, a number in excess of the total number of paid staff in those sectors. Many volunteers are small social institutions in themselves, like lollipop men and women, bureaucratically known as school crossing patrol officers or school crossing wardens, who have a daily partnership with parents and children to keep them as safe as possible from the risk of road traffic accidents.

Volunteering is a major element of modern citizen participation, and has been for decades, boosted by programmes like Help a London Child, Comic Relief and Children in Need. Volunteering is generally enjoyable, whether the volunteer is a student or an older person, and one survey reported 100 per cent of volunteering learners rated the experience as beneficial (Deepak and Wallace 2008).

In the last decade, traditional volunteering, based on loose affiliations of volunteers overseen by a management committee, has evolved into a service similar to those in the paid sectors characterised by a 'professionalisation of volunteer management, with an emphasis on quality standards and accreditation of volunteers' (Kearney 2001). This has partly been a response

Community organisations providing mainstream social care services

For the first time ever, in the 1990s, five state agencies in Missouri, USA, put together a cross-agency budget of $21.6 million, to improve services to children and families, and involved families directly in the process through a series of community partnerships known as the Missouri Partners Group. This changed how the state government and communities worked together. Other states like Vermont, Oregon and Maryland subsequently did the same.

Each community in Missouri was given a budget to form its own community collaborative, particularly to develop new community leaders. After four years, improved outcomes included lower levels of suspension from school, improvements in academic performance, and far more accessible local services (Rozansky 1997).

In the UK, Keeping House, Angels Housekeeping and HOPS (Hawksworth Older Peoples Support) are community-based social enterprises, supported by Leeds City Council, providing services such as shopping, domestic services, gardening, cleaning and small repairs for the elderly and disabled, encouraging local people to take up this as a social enterprise.

These community social and business partnerships incorporate a range of interventions and aim at improving outcomes at the social, community educational and employment levels, rather than one intervention and one outcome at a time.

to the contract culture and the requirements of funders that volunteers be screened before starting, and supervised on their tasks.

Volunteers can form partnerships with service users even in the most complex cases and in the most high-profile service areas like child protection. For example, CSV developed their Volunteers in Child Protection (ViCP) programme, in which trained and supported volunteers work alongside local authority social workers to increase trust between the families and professionals. The pilot projects, run in two local authorities, were independently evaluated (Tunstill 2007).

The ViCP project was found to be successful at recruiting and preparing volunteers to work with complex needs. With the appropriate preparation, they were well able to undertake child protection work, undaunted by the range of challenging circumstances of the families they met. Although the size of the sample was limited, the study found evidence of positive outcomes for both children and their parents. For example, a family where the parents were once reluctant to engage with social workers was now doing so. For instance, the improvement in a mother's self-esteem enabled her to begin to get her own life back on track, by volunteering as a classroom assistant at her child's school, and contemplating an NVQ qualification.

However the study also underlined important messages for social work and social care organizations in respect of prioritising the offer of support at the earliest possible stage, to forestall later problems developing. The project officers were crucial to the viability and success of the scheme and their location in the respective children's services departments maximized the chances of eliciting referrals from social workers. The positive attitude and role of managers was similarly pivotal and could signal to the staff they managed, the importance of making extra support available to those families who need it. In reality, multiple partnerships are essential if any small project is to get off the ground.

Volunteers are now major partners in every profession. Special constables have some of the powers of police officers, and are ordinary working people volunteering on top of their day job up to a maximum of 16 hours a month. A volunteering scheme for university students is in place in return for a reduction in tuition fees. Permanent disaster volunteers, supported by organisations like the Red Cross, are available round the clock in the event of any UK disaster, and are always rapidly mobilised, working together with the statutory emergency services. In all these examples, volunteers contribute significant social capital to society.

Paid social work grew out of volunteering. The timeline goes back through generations of altruistic individuals, forming an invisible national network from at least the middle ages onwards, including major contributions to war efforts.

Today's volunteers divide between those who can only spare a short amount of time, fitting volunteering into busy lives, and those, particularly retired people, for whom volunteering can become a full-time activity, whether in a high street charity shop, mentoring a vulnerable child or adult, or acting as the unpaid treasurer on the board of a large charity. Many so-called para-professionals are essentially volunteers as the pay they receive only covers a fraction of their costs if the time they spend is fully taken into account. Hustinx makes a distinction between 'classic volunteering', which is more stable and inspired by collective identities and traditional roles, and 'new volunteering', which is a matter of personal preferences (Hustinx 2001). An example of new volunteering was the arrival of 30,000 spontaneous and unaffiliated volunteers at the World Trade Center after the September 11 terrorist attacks in New York in 2001.

Volunteering has diversified in the last decade with many partnership organisations starting up, such as the National Council for Black Volunteering, the Millennium Volunteers Programme, Futurebuilders, the National Centre for Volunteering and Active Community initiatives. The private sector has also started to provide volunteers to meet corporate social responsibility targets and obligations. For example, Barclays Bank has enabled thousands of its employees to volunteer for its partnership project with NCH called

'Financial Futures', to provide financial workshops to NCH service users on issues such as dealing with a debt crisis.

Volunteering has also been repeatedly eulogised by successive governments, who have linked it strongly to community capacity building and place shaping (see Chapter 2). Volunteering has a number of intrinsic merits and spin offs. In a study of voluntary work in Tanzania, Naryan demonstrated a link between involvement in volunteering and household welfare (Naryan 1999). Several policy reviews, such as the Russell Commission on Youth Volunteering, have resulted in development funding and expansionist programmes. On the ground, this has translated into more support for volunteers and more training opportunities.

However, lest this sound too rosy, a key question is whether the care workers and volunteers of the future will be there?

In 2006, Marjorie Covey, aged 84, retired from running the Northfield Centre luncheon club in Wellington, Somerset, after 21 years service for the WRVS. The club serves 120 meals a week, and is a source of social care support for vulnerable local people. No one has come forward yet to keep the centre going (*Wellington Weekly News*, 19 July 2006). The WRVS is an example of a trusted organisation which from time to time needs to renew itself. It has 2,500 staff and 70,000 volunteers. Polls show the public thinks of it as 'trusted, reliable and kind'. In the same week, Seaton Youth Centre announced it would be forced to close in August 2006 because no new volunteers came forward after the existing group of volunteer trustees decided to call it a day after 14 years (www.midweekherald.co.uk, also 19 July 2006). There are grounds for cautious optimism in the numbers of retired people living longer and coming forward to volunteer, also in large numbers, but however good a resource volunteers are, they cannot be taken for granted.

Partnerships with philanthropists

For more than three millennia, regardless of society or culture, the history of philanthropy has seen a minute percentage of personal or corporate wealth flowing to 'good causes' – centuries of support for 'the deserving poor'. My wife's maternal grandfather, a hosiery manufacturer in Wigston, Leicestershire who made the first football socks in the UK, funded a baby welfare service run by his wife in the town. Genuine acts of kindness and tolerance are commonplace, even in the midst of great hostility. At the outset of the Australian colony, English jailers began to soften their regime for the convicts they were brutalising, partly through the realisation that the convicts were becoming settlers and a new colony could not be developed as a countrywide prison (Keneally 1968). Even in the most punitive regimes and times, the importance of rehabilitation stares everyone involved in the face.

Today, charity giving is more commercialised. Businesses such as chemical companies and banks will normally now give a small percentage of their profits to good causes through their own arms-length foundations, often with the triple intention of softening their image and demonstrating corporate social responsibility: advertising the business; and leaving a legacy locally, through funding a service or a building for example. Sainsbury's works with organisations like Mencap to give work experience and apprenticeships to young people with learning disabilities, and also expressed interest in a scheme to offer careers to young people in the care system, in a national community business partnership, just as HSBC is funding private tutors for children in care in four pilot local authorities. Oxfam receives an annual £1 million contract for providing volunteers at the Glastonbury Festival.

Charities compete with each other to persuade customers in busy shopping centres, out to spend money on something else, to divert a small percentage their way. Cold selling has become professionalised, so trained sellers from larger charities will stand alongside committed volunteers coming out on behalf of small charities who depend far more on street donations for survival. Cold calling is commonplace, including door knocking. Social care is no longer exempt from the hard sell culture.

Despite the risk of donation fatigue from a surfeit of direct requests for money, fundraising events, and increased competition for patronage, large sums can be raised or secured through donations. Increasing wealth in the UK means huge contributions can, with a combination of luck and skill, be levered in from corporate or private sources. The NSPCC Fresh Start Centre for action on child sexual abuse is based in a building in Camden, north London, converted with a £10 million donation by the property tycoon, Richard Caring, who soon after bought the Mayfair night club, Annabel's. The Sainsbury Foundation gives the National Children's Bureau over £1 million each year. Centrica partnered with Help the Aged in 1999 and by 2004 had raised £4.5 million. Two charitable trusts, Ark, chaired by the hedge fund millionaire Arpad Busson, and the Edtrust Foundation, chaired by a prominent local businessman, Lord Amir Bhatia, are taking charge of and sponsoring four secondary schools in Birmingham, planning to turn two of them into new City Academies. Roger De Haan, founder of Saga Holidays, is putting over £40 million of investment into the establishment of a new university for Folkestone, echoing the benevolence of a seventeenth-century philanthropist, the cloth merchant John Harrison (1579–1656) who, as the co-founder of the Leeds Corporation, endowed the city-to-be with almshouses and a grammar school.

Philanthropy is no longer the exclusive province of the rich. In that sense, philanthropy has been democratised, with millions of employees giving to charity through payroll donations, to support diverse causes such as adopting animals in London Zoo – paying for an animal's annual feed by direct debit – or perhaps by sponsoring a child in need overseas. A Docklands special school (the Stephen Hawking School) received an anonymous donation of £10,000 to help with renovations, and a parent, Annabel Goodman, backed by Adam Cresswell, bought the New Elizabethan School autistic school in

A year in the planning, a night in the making

The charity which I chair, BAAF, held a gala dinner on 28 February 2008 for nearly 400 guests, at the Park Lane Hotel in London, to raise money for its work on behalf of children in care. The dinner took a year to plan, led by Dinner Committee co-chairs, Annabel Elliott, a well-known interior designer, and Andrew Last, MD of a global PR company. A host of celebrities such as Jemima Khan, Lenny Henry and Nicky Campbell came to support the charity. On the night, over £150,000 was raised, after deducting costs, through auctioning donated prizes like luxury holidays, a dinner party in your own home cooked by a celebrity chef and backstage passes to rock concerts – partnership working with the generous and affluent on the night.

Celebrity support for the work of charities is crucial for them to achieve the necessary profile for attracting publicity and the funds that go with it, like Martin Clunes (Macmillan Cancer Relief); Cat Deeley, and Ant and Dec (Great Ormond Street Children's Charity); and Graham Norton (Marie Curie Cancer Care).

the Worcestershire village of Hartlebury because she opposed its closure and did not want her son to be put back into state education.

The pastoral work of religious groups is part of this tradition. Joseph and Benjamin Seebohm Rowntree, the York-born Quaker chocolate entrepreneurs, built the village of New Eastwick to provide affordable housing for their workers. In the Second World War, Quakers helped Jews from Austria flee their homeland to the safety of England. Today, Quakers are working in Palestine, re-homing families under threat.

Just as the number of informal carers was widely under-estimated until recently, the numbers of citizens making a contribution through contemporary philanthropy runs into the millions, and that is without the contribution of everyone buying a National Lottery ticket, or participating in Sport Relief activities, many of the proceeds for which go to supporting vulnerable people.

Some giving is in the form of sponsorship and publicity, not financial help, like the Beat the Bully campaign in southeast London, supported by Charlton Athletic Football Club. Alan Curbishley, then Charlton Athletic manager, wrote to Thomas Tallis School, saying 'With regard to the "Beat Bully" wristbands, I have given them to the team captain, Matt Holland, who will put them in the team's dressing room for the players to wear at their discretion'. Most of the players did, for the next few games, in front of thousands of fans.

Partnerships with philanthropists are fundamentally about a process of connection between a charity and its potential funders, whereby a chord is

Philanthropy within children's services

Brighton and Hove Children's Trust supports the Soundmakers Programme, which aims to give every child in every primary school in Brighton and Hove a musical instrument and free tuition from a local musician – Brighton being blessed with many. A government grant covers most of the costs of tuition but not the cost of the many and varied instruments children wish to learn. Cherito Jones, owner of Momma Cherri's restaurant in Brighton, leads a fundraising programme to meet these costs, based upon asking everyone who eats at a participating restaurant in Brighton to make a voluntary donation to the fund of £1 when settling their bill. A similar initiative is Jail Guitar Doors, a creative rehabilitation scheme championed by the musician Billy Bragg to provide prison inmates with access to musical instruments.

The importance of partnership working with musicians in children's social care is also illustrated by the contributions made by the chairman of the Brighton Youth Orchestra to local discussions about information sharing in child protection cases, which he felt were needed on the basis that many children confide in their music teacher.

struck and a commitment is nurtured. The search process is going on every minute of every day, through appeals on national and local radio, through social networking, word of mouth, poster advertising and intranet sites – new partnerships in waiting.

Partnerships with the media

Social care issues have moved from the media margin to mainstream primetime programming in a constant bombardment of the viewing public with social issues, especially in soaps like *EastEnders*. In any single week, dramas or documentaries about vulnerable children or adults now provide routine entertainment. Programmes reflect the complexity of issues facing people compared to a generation ago. The 2007 BBC drama, *Stuart: A Life Backwards*, showed the reasons a young man was homeless and why he eventually took his own life (Masters 2005). His background contained sibling violence, bullying, physical abuse by his father, sexual abuse by the notorious Cambridge care home paedophile, Keith Laverack, as well as an underlying physical condition, muscular dystrophy. In the influential 1966 drama, *Cathy Come Home*, the sole issue was the brutality of a public service that took children into care solely because their parents were homeless, with no other social problems (Sandford 1967).

The explosion of interest in social care means all social care agencies and professionals need to be media-savvy, so that they feed good news stories to the media, to balance the inevitable occasional bad news. The media is in part a check and balance on misused professional power, and 'new public journalism' in which anyone can have their say by sending in their stories, or through phone-ins, can lead to a partnership between the media and people who use services, to expose poor levels of service. That so little is made of this is partly a sign that the majority of service provision falls within an acceptable range, and partly a sign of service user disempowerment, through fear, lack of awareness and the digital divide.

The media can help or destroy in equal proportion. Whilst negative stories about social care far outweigh positive coverage, and when a film company in Nottingham can bribe young people to act as young homeless as one did, *The Sun* prints pictures and sensitive profiles of children needing families during National Adoption Week every year, supporting the drive to find permanent caring homes for children in care in the UK. The media is a fact of life – and a key partnership to put time and effort into for a profession often under fire. Of course it is wrong to think of the media as solely the print media, and solely the national print media at that. Many local newspapers and the social care trade press work in a positive partnership with the social care profession and agencies, printing thousands of informative and positive stories every year. And the media has an impact. The NSPCC online advice site for children and young people, There4me.com, normally has four young people in the queue for a service. Within two minutes of a brief feature about the programme on a lunchtime chat show, the number waiting went up to 80.

A tale of three women: how the media helped to raise the profile of the carer's movement

The carer's movement grew from invisibility to global recognition within 25 years, partly through a partnership with the media to highlight an issue that affects one in six people in the UK, particularly women. The movement started with the campaigning zeal of two carers. The Rev Mary Webster gave up her work as a minister in 1954, when she was 31, to look after her parents, later founding the National Council for the Single Woman and her Dependents. Judith Oliver looked after her disabled husband and founded the Association of Carers in 1981. To gain the highest profile possible, turning private stress and despair into a public issue, it had to develop a single voice, and to become an unbreachable alliance. Jill Pitkeathley, now Baroness Pitkeathley, merged the two organisations in 1988 to form the Carers National Association, now Carers UK.

The movement's milestones were incremental legislative gains. The Invalid Care Allowance was extended to married women in 1986. The Carers Recognition and Services Act 1995 gave carers the right to an assessment of their own needs, and not just the needs of the person they were caring for, and even if the cared-for person refused to be assessed. The Carers and Disabled Children Act 2000, and the Carers (Equal Opportunities) Act 2004, extended the right to services to new groups, in measures such as enabling local authorities to provide carers with vouchers for breaks, ensuring that carers are informed of their rights, that work, lifelong learning and leisure are considered when a carer is assessed, and giving local authorities new powers to enlist the help of housing, health, education and other public bodies in providing support to carers.

Jill Pitkeathley became known as the media Martini girl, getting the media on her side to draw public attention to the plight of carers, partly through always having a carer ready and waiting to be interviewed. Her media strategy was to come up with some 'sledgehammer' facts, such as – 'there are six million carers in the UK, about one in seven of the population, saving the Treasury £34 billion'. A partnership with statisticians at the Family Policy Studies Centre supported the campaigns. The statistics were good for soundbites and led to a big increase in fundraising. The movement worked through an alliance, the Carers Alliance, bringing in other organisations to become as formidable as possible when dealing with government ministers and officials. They engaged key politicians like Malcolm Wicks, another carers champion, in building vital cross-party support. This culminated in the launch of the National Carers Strategy by the then Prime Minister, Tony Blair, in 1999.

The six principles of the Carers Alliance are:

- Be united, make common cause
- Be prepared to compromise and negotiate
- Stay politically neutral
- Be patient
- Be aware there is always more to do
- Never miss an opportunity.

For the media as a whole, the carers movement is part of the acceptable face of social care. The less acceptable side receives far more coverage, including the more damaging headline coverage of supposed miscarriages of justice, failure to protect vulnerable people, or would-be adopters frustrated by bureaucrats. The issue here is what the media defines as good, worthy or acceptable, which often depends on the spin put on a story rather than the facts.

Even prominent social care journalists can have their positive pieces scuppered by desk editors' preference for the negative, salacious or sensational. After it was repeatedly left out of the paper, David Brindle, *The Guardian*'s public services editor, gave up attempting to place a story he had written about the remarkable popularity of the first personal budgets in social care, even though their success presaged a sea change in the way public services are organised and delivered (personal discussion). Reputations suffer from adverse media coverage, particularly stereotyping, or gratuitous asides such as one in a pop novel – 'All the pen pushers from the council are coming' he replied, 'and the busybodies from social services' (Haran 2002).

Public opinion does change over time. MORI found that in March 1990, the big issues facing Britain were the poll tax (49 per cent); inflation (26 per cent); the NHS (25 per cent); and economy (24 per cent). By 2003, with the poll tax abolished and inflation at much lower levels, the five biggest issues were defence (64 per cent), the NHS (35 per cent), education (27 per cent), crime (21 per cent) and the economy (12 per cent) (Ipsos MORI). At the time of writing, social care is undoubtedly moving higher up the agenda, partly due to the cumulative impact and exposure of so many high-profile partnership programmes. This includes the first Government-led recruitment advertisements for jobs in social care on national television.

The medium is the message (McLuhan 1967), and this can include use of all available media – see the BAAF poster campaign, Figure 4.1, to highlight the plight of children in the care system who are moved around. Over the course of a week in 2006, the posters were moved around major cities, becoming more frayed, symbolically, in the process.

Many information sheets and internal training videos could and would be used by local or regional media with a more proactive media strategy. The opportunity to work more positively with the media to gain coverage for the positive work being done across social care remains seriously untapped, and is an argument for investing in a strong media and communications team inside agencies or across an alliance of organisations. However, the uphill task facing communication professionals attempting to place good news stories about social care is illustrated by the fact that when Bradford Council put up posters boasting of the amount it was spending on children in the care system, the overwhelming local reaction was horror at the amount, not praise for the investment being made.

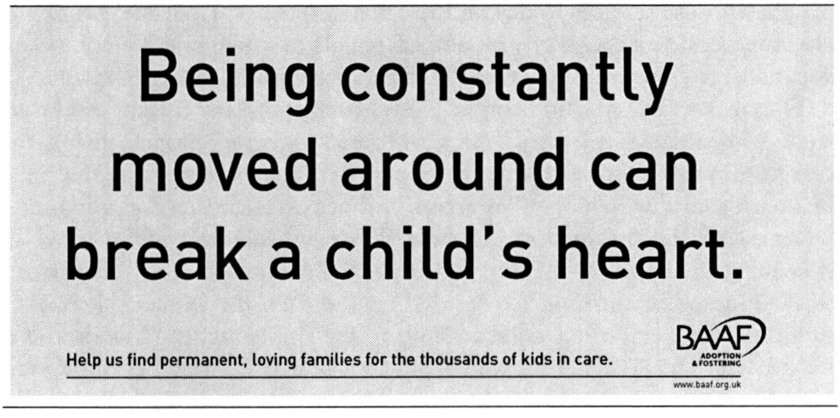

Being constantly moved around can break a child's heart.

Help us find permanent, loving families for the thousands of kids in care.

BAAF
ADOPTION & FOSTERING
www.baaf.org.uk

Figure 4.1 BAAF poster

Partnerships with artists

This section of my book may not appear immediately relevant to the issues about partnership working in social care, but I am seeking to illustrate the power of art, music, theatre and dance to support people who use services directly, and to inspire staff to think of ways they can use art in the broadest sense in their work.

By changing and challenging the way reality is perceived, artists can stimulate different ways of thinking, which is a central theme of partnership working. In his work *Constellations* (77 million paintings), Brian Eno, the ex-Roxy Music guitarist, digitised 300 paintings through a software programme which generated and projected constantly evolving paintings onto a screen – it would take several million years to witness all the possible 77 million combinations the software can create. This is also a metaphor for partnership working, particularly complex multiple partnerships, which are constantly evolving, with new people coming in, and others leaving (installation at the Baltic Centre for Contemporary Art, Gateshead, 2007).

Artists change the way an object is looked at and thought about, such as the Australian sculptor Ron Muerck's larger than life-size sculptures of people of all ages, from huge babies to tiny old people. The French artist Louise Bourgeois built a cell with her house inside it, with a guillotine hanging over the house, symbolising the constant risk of family violence. Artists like Andy Warhol and Keith Haring fundamentally redefined the artist's relationship with the general public, shifting art from an exclusive group of insiders, to public property in a much more commercialised and interactive way. Direct engagement with the public requires much stronger partnership values and 'virtue ethics' (Allison 2005). Many artists with these values work directly with people who use services in day and residential services. Collaborative artists like Anna Best work with groups of local people in situ in real-life events and situations, to transform how those involved perceive their environment.

Film makers like Martin Scorsese, Ken Loach and many theatre producers work with a group of actors on a 'working together' model, giving the cast freedom to interpret the script or play as it comes to mind at the time, in Loach's case with unknown actors and actresses chosen for bringing a freshness to the production. Scorsese illustrates this evolving method in describing his work in his film *The Departed* 'Nicholson [Jack Nicholson] worked in a different way. We decided on the date, the age and the power of his character, and the fact he's falling apart. This is the way I work, this is my process. The other actors can talk, but we all worked together' (interview with Martin Scorsese in *Epoch Times*, 28 March–3 April 2007).

Art facilitates personal expression, and through that supports vulnerable people, even inside high security institutions with maximum containment and little stimulation. Art is a mainstream activity in many community projects and programmes, especially day care. Painting, music and drama projects can bring groups of service users together across boundaries to showcase

---

'I don't do anything really'

During a team meeting with a local community learning disability team, when I was a Director of Social Services, I asked all team members what their interests and passions were and how they might best express them in their work. The team administrator said, 'I don't do anything really'. When pressed, she said, almost confidingly, that her passion was bell ringing. She rang the church bells in her local village and sometimes in surrounding villages on special occasions. She was an expert bell-ringer. The outcome was that from then on she spent half a day every week in a bell-ringing session with people with severe learning disabilities, which was built into the activity programmes of three local day centres, and gave many people who used those services great pleasure.

---

their abilities. Many staff have unexpressed skills which can be built into programmes to support people who use services (see 'I don't do anything really' box above).

Art needs its partnership workers too. *Flourish* is a project initiated by the London Borough of Newham and supported by a number of organisations such as PricewaterhouseCoopers, the Government Office for London, and PIPC, highlighting the artwork of children looked after in the UK. Its curator, Beatty Hallas, puts on exhibitions around the UK for artists whose search, as she puts it, 'is for a place to be' (Flourish 2006). One exhibitor, Danny Wortington, said 'I am 17 years old, and I've been in care for six years. I have been able to express myself and have grown in confidence through my photos. It is my main interest and passion. With my camera I am able to look at life in a different way. When I pick up a camera, I feel great. Every time I use my camera I learn something new' (Flourish 2006).

Artistic techniques can be used in training and development programmes. For example, use of split screen filming, showing different stories, or different aspects of the same story, simultaneously on screen – can illustrate what different family members, or members of a partnership team are thinking on the same issue. Lower costs of digital filming can mean high-quality DVDs and print material can be produced quickly to a high standard without always using expensive professional commissions – *Life and Deaf* is an innovative speech and language therapy project involving severely and profoundly deaf children aged 6–19. They produced a DVD and book of poetry which was distributed widely in Greenwich, southeast London. A 15-year-old deaf poet commented 'I feel proud of it and my parents are proud too'.

Drama also has its place in promoting partnership working. *A Change of Mind* was a play staged in Sadlers Wells which used the views of Islington Council's own staff about their borough's change programme, which was aimed at changing the way they thought about their jobs and delivered their services. Key opinions from staff were integrated into the drama, such as:

- On motivation: 'how can I be motivated when I've been in the same job for ten years?'
- On consultation: 'it's all a paper exercise'
- On customer focus: 'are we serving the organisation or the customer?'
- Cynicism: 'we've seen it all before'
- Management style: 'them and us'
- Equality and responsibility: 'different rules for different troops'
- Leadership: 'lead by example'.

The play reflected back to staff their own cynicism and the impact this had on those around them, which was followed up by the council in local development programmes. The council also acknowledged the need to change some of its operating practices which were partly responsible for the alienation.

Drama strategies can also help vulnerable people express themselves and tuition or classes can be built into a care plan (Baldwin 2004). The film star Thandie Newton started out with a scholarship from Cornwall County Council to train as a dancer. The history of staged drama is full of classic partnerships, like Portia and Nerissa's mission to save Antonio in Shakespeare's *The Merchant of Venice*, which also featured the memorable lines by Shylock about being Jewish in Elizabethan England, in a key speech about diversity which any victim of discrimination down the ages would echo:

> Hath not a Jew eyes? Hath not a Jew hands, organs, dimensions, senses, affections, passions?

A voluntary group, Dance United, uses dance training as a frontline youth justice service in Bradford, and the films of Pedro Almodovar all show intensely unique networks of people, often made up of superficially like-minded individuals who have met each other by chance

Music and literature can be inspirational for social workers. Books like *The Curious Incident of the Dog in the Night-Time*, about how a 15-year-old boy with autism, encouraged by a social worker at school to record his investigations, tries to find out who killed his neighbour's dog (Haddon 2004). A colleague of mine, whose oldest son is on the autistic spectrum, says her younger son understood much more about his older brother having read this book, especially the unavoidable and unintentional hard-wired challenging behaviour that can accompany autism. A study by the Social Workers Education Trust found that social care staff found many other books inspirational in their work (SWET 2006).

Much great music has strong sociaanl care themes, which can be used to increase awareness in training programmes. Janacek's opera, *Jenufa*, is about the inner conflicts of a foster child. Puccini's opera, *Madam Butterfly*, is a tragic story of an inter-country adoption and the impact of the loss of her child on a Japanese birth mother. Donizetti's opera *Lucia di Lammermoor* tells the story of forcing a young woman into a marriage she does not want, after which she kills her husband and goes mad. Steve Reich's (music) and Beryl Korot's (video) partnership in film and music *Hindenburg + Bikini + Dolly*, shows how contemporary events in the public mind can be contextualised through different pairs of eyes. Subtle partnerships can also be expressed through music. The third movement of Shostakovich's Tenth Symphony features a tune within a tune: within the thundering socialist realist soundscape is a lilting tune representing the hidden, discreet partnership between Shostakovich and Elmira Nazirova, his Azeri composition pupil, who was also 'his muse, confidante and object of unrequited affection at the time' (programme notes to Valery Gergiev's Shostakovich cycle at the Barbican, 2006).

Partnership champions

Tens of thousands of inspirational individuals in all walks of life make a contribution to civic society, and who, as a result, are in a supportive partnership with great numbers of people whose lives they touch and influence. In China, such people are known as 'can do commanders'.

- Steve Evans is a paramedic with 34 years in the Emergency Ambulance Service and the founder of the Don't Walk Away campaign. He organises poster campaigns and speaks at conferences to promote citizen responsibility for vulnerable people.
- Deborah Howe is a champion of children and young people in Leeds. She manages the Project West Yorkshire Youth Association, and has been nominated to be the first children and young people's involvement advocate. She campaigned to set up a children and young people's charter, and worked with young people from Beeston and Woodhouse so they could have their say after the 7/7 bombings in 2005.
- Since 1966, John Wade, a councillor in Barnsley, has campaigned to get the River Don cleaned up, after it was polluted by an old mine works. Finally in 1998, with the help of £470,000 EU cash, a new £1.2 million scheme began to pump out the waste.
- Margaret Harrison set up the first Home-start service – a peer support service for new parents – in 1973. By 2007, there were 345 schemes and 15,000 trained parent volunteers (Harrison 2003). Today there are large number of such peer support services, including good parent-to-parent communication mediated by specialist websites such as the one set up by Parentline Plus (www.parentlineplus.org.uk).
- Julie Wright, a Norfolk mother whose 16-year-old son Steven was killed when he crossed the A148 between Fakenham and Holt, successfully campaigned for Norfolk County Council to cut the speed limit on the fatal stretch from 60 to 40 mph and to put in pedestrian refuges.

- The relatives of Victoria Climbié, through the Victoria Climbié Foundation, work with groups of African women on issues like child trafficking, and with African faith groups on safeguarding issues, particularly to make sure that 'other African children who make this journey (to England)' are kept safe.
- David Yorke died at 85 on 4 January 2007 in Needham Market, Suffolk. After he retired in 1981, he opened a charity shop at the Museum of East Anglian Life in Stowmarket, raising more than £40,000. He was Chair of Governors at a local school, President of the local Horticultural Society, active in the British Legion, and for 21 years was one of a team distributing meals on wheels locally.
- Barnaby Blackburn is a 12-year-old dyslexic boy who developed a unique partnership with the Apple Corporation who sponsored his website (www.iamdyslexic.com) inspiring other young people with dyslexia to be more confident.

Mrs Cline and Ms Modi

Evelyn Cline is white and in her eighties. Ayesha Modi is British Asian and 18. The link between them is that they were, respectively, the first and the most recent Youth Mayors for Southend in Essex. In the early 1950s, the first youth workers and youth representatives in the UK came together, through the National Youth Conference. Mrs Cline ran the monthly youth ball in Southend, which raised money for the café, which served hot chocolate, and which was where the youth of Southend could hang out. The ball, held on Southend Pier, had a live band and the boys in that era wore dinner suits. In her role as Youth Mayor, Mrs Cline remembers going to tea with Princess Margaret and the Archbishop of Canterbury at Lambeth Palace after the Coronation of Queen Elizabeth II in 1953.

Ms Modi, the Youth Mayor in 2006/7, was funded through the local Connexions partnership. She still represents Southend youth at local events, but focuses on getting things done, often issuing press releases to draw public attention to issues. One has been to break up the tension between gangs of local Chavs, Goths and Polepaks, hanging around Southend town centre. She also sits on various council committees, scrutiny panels and boards, and works with local MPs in Essex on a Youth Politics Group. Her spell as Youth Mayor has confirmed for her that she wants to go into politics.

Both women say it was an honour to be Youth Mayor and to serve the youth community, then and now.

Davina James Hanman

Hidden Histories is a guide to plaques in the London Borough of Camden dedicated to women like Millicent Garret Fawcett, who championed womens suffrage; Mary Wollstonecraft and Beatrice Webb, both pioneering advocates for the rights of women; and Marie Stopes, Jacqueline Du Pré and Christina Rossetti, to name but a few. Davina James Hanman does not have her own plaque, but if there is any justice in years to come, she will. Like Erin Pizzey a decade before her, she has campaigned for the last 20 years to raise awareness of the pervasive and widespread impact of domestic violence on women in relationships and in families. Her work programme includes training front line staff like police officers, speaking at seminars and conferences, and directly supporting staff in individual women's refuges. Her knowledge of the subject is typical of single-issue, driven people. As she says herself, 'I forget my own birthday but I remember everything about domestic violence. Violence against women is a major cost to women themselves and to society. Social care services spends millions on it indirectly with little publicity because it is a secondary issue'.

Davina first became interested in counselling women whilst at university in Norwich, but she had actually been campaigning since she was nine or ten years old for one cause or another, fired up by a sense of social injustice. She worked in women's centres, took part in Reclaim the Night marches organised after two late-night stranger rapes in Norwich, and drove tourist camper trucks across Africa, all before she was 25. By then, she knew she wanted a lifelong career in the womens' movement, an aspiration made more complicated by the closure of one women's unit after another in the early 1990s, as British local authorities asset-stripped their equal opportunities infrastructures, optimistically claiming that gender-sensitive approaches were by then thoroughly incorporated into the mainstream of organisations. She says she is 'glad someone pays me to be obsessed'. That someone is a combination of trust funds, the Mayor of London and a wide variety of statutory agencies and partnerships who commission work from Davina and her team. She wants to grow from being the voice of domestic violence in London to being a national and then an international voice for women victims, possibly through the United Nations. She cites low-cost housing projects with integrated job training for women in India, and new grass roots women's organisations in Brazil, as examples of how in many ways the developing world is the place to be for radical women these days. Above all else, Davina James Hanman illustrates how much one person can achieve on their own, despite being faced with hostility from vested interests, and held back by a chronic long-term lack of funding and bureaucratic obstacles.

Countless individuals have developed new partnership services, campaigning for decades (see the boxes above). Many such partnerships have their origins in chance encounters or in a dynamic conversation. Gill Haworth, the inter-country adoption pioneer, started work as an adoption worker in Tower Hamlets in 1971, then became a team leader in family placement services, then a specialist inter-country adoption worker. Between 1997 and 2001, she met with a group of like-minded professionals around her kitchen table, which led to the formation of the Overseas Adoption Helpline, later to become the Inter-country Adoption Centre. They went on to help develop government guidance, and to run preparation courses for inter-country adopters co-facilitated by an adoptive parent and an adoption worker.

And last but not least, your own partnership network

Partnership working is a personal responsibility for all social care professionals. The question each professional in each separate agency should ask themselves is not whether partnership working is applicable but: *what is the partnership I need to be a part of or to lead in this case or in this situation?* – defined by Hornby and Atkins as 'the minimum essential collaboration' (Hornby and Atkins 1993).

As well as this, each individual practitioner and manager in social care has their own partnership network, made up of family members, friends, and present or ex-colleagues who are trusted, who inspire, who are loyal, reliable, supportive and understanding. A close colleague of mine who narrowly escaped death from cancer keeps in touch with the surgeon who saved her life. The surgeon in turn derives personal and professional pride and pleasure from seeing her patient's achievements. This is an example of how personal and professional partnerships can't always be kept separate, nor should they necessarily be.

My current partnerships at work

I work with a board of 12 members in my day job and chair a board of the same number in a national voluntary organisation. In the former, I work with 150 managers, and in the latter, about 20. I have around 50 crucial external partnerships without which I could not do my job. I also have less direct partnerships with staff at all levels, and with a range of contacts inside and outside my organisation(s). This adds up to approximately 200 significant partnerships and 1,000 'occasional partnerships' to maintain. Whatever the level you work at in social care, you will probably be in a partnership of some description with between 100 and 800 people, be they service users, relatives or professionals. That is the reality of partnership working and networking today!

A career in social care can be emotionally draining and physically challenging, as well as being a great privilege – 'the loneliness of the long-distance social worker'. Workers need to be near to 100 per cent fit, physically and psychologically, to keep going. Support inside work is one thing, and vital, but so is support outside work through your own personal relationship and networks. The Doctors Support Network, formed in a partnership with the charity PriMHE, has a support line, a monthly newsletter and an email forum for distressed doctors (www.primhe.org). Social care workers are the unrecognised fourth emergency service, intervening during a crisis in lives at breaking point. Strong personal and professional networks are often the only reason why social care staff are able to keep going, year in, year out.

References

Allison, A., 2005, 'Ethical issues of working in partnership', in R. Carnwell and J. Buchanan (eds), *Effective Practice in Health and Social Care: A Partnership Approach*, Buckingham: Open University Press.

Balbernie, R., 2007, 'Circuits and circumstances: the neurobiological consequences of early relationships', *Judicial Studies Board: Journal of Child Psychotherapy*, 27(3): 237–55.

Baldwin, P., 2004, *With Drama in Mind*, Stafford: Network Educational Press.

Cairns, B., Harris, M. and Carrol, M., 2006, 'Professional researchers in the community', in R. Cnaan and C. Milofsky (eds), *Handbook of Community Movements and Local Organisations*, New York: Kluwer/Plenum Press.

Community Care, 2006, 'A seamless transition', 21 September.

Deepak, S. and Wallace, E., 2008, *Assessing the Impact of Volunteering on the Further Education Sector*, London: Volunteering England.

Flourish, 2006, *2006 Catalogue*, London: London Borough of Newham Children's Services.

Greater London Authority, 2006, *Towards Joined-up Lives: Disabled and Deaf Londoners' Experience of Housing, Employment and Post-16 Education from a Social Model Perspective*, London: Greater London Authority.

Haddon, M., 2004, *The Curious Incident of the Dog in the Night-time*, London: Vintage.

Haran, M., 2002, *Husband Material*, London: Little, Brown.

Harrison, M., 2003, *Hooray! Here Comes Tuesday: The Home-Start Story*, Leicester: Bamaha Publishing.

Henwood, M. and Hudson, B., 2007, *Here to Stay? Self-directed Support: Aspiration and Implementation*, London: Department of Health.

Hornby, S. and Atkins, J., 1993, *Collaborative Care: Inter-professional, Inter-agency and Interpersonal*, Oxford: Blackwell.

Hustinx, L., 2001, 'Individualisation and new styles of youth volunteering: an empirical explanation', *Voluntary Action*, 3(2): 57–76.

Kearney, J., 2001, The values and basic principles of volunteering: complacency or caution?, *Voluntary Action*, 3(3): 63–86.

Keneally, T., 1968, *Bring Larks and Heroes*, London: Viking Penguin.

Lisenburgh, S. and Harding, R., 2000, *Knowledge Links: Innovation in University/ Business Partnerships*, London: Institute for Public Policy Research.

Masters, A., 2005, *Stuart: A Life Backwards*, London: HarperPerennial.

McCrystal, P. and Godfrey, A., 2001, 'Developing a researcher–practitioner partnership for the effective evaluation of professional social work training', *Social Work Education*, 20(5): 539–49.

McLuhan, M., 1967, *The Medium is the Message*, New York: Bantam.

Naryan, D., 1999, *Complementarity and Substitution: Social Capital, Poverty Reduction and the State*, The Environmentally and Socially Sustainable Development Studies and Monographs Series No 20, Washington, DC: World Bank.

Rozansky, P., 1997, *Missourians Working Together: A Progress Report*, Jefferson City, MO: Family Investment Trust.

Sandford, J., 1967, *Cathy Come Home*, Harmondsworth: Penguin (also BBC DVD, 2003).

SCIE, 2006, *The Learning, Teaching and Assessment of Partnership Work in Social Work Education*, Knowledge Review 10, London: SCIE.

Social Workers Educational Trust (SWET), 2006, *Be Inspired; Social Work Literary Influences*, Birmingham: SWET.

Thoburn, J., 2007, 'Review of research and other sources of knowledge relevant to the fostering service provided to these children and their foster carers', in B. Parrott, A. MacIver and J. Thoburn, *Independent Inquiry Report into the Circumstances of Child Sexual Abuse by Two Foster Carers in 2007*, Wakefield: Wakefield Council.

Tucker, S., Hughes, J., Scott, J. and Challis, D., 2007, 'Commissioning services for older people with mental health problems: is there a shared vision?' *Journal of Integrated Care*, 15(2): 3–12.

Tunstill, J., 2007, *The Volunteers in Child Protection Project: Early Evaluation Findings*, London: CSV, London.

UK Inquiry into Mental Health and Well-Being in Later life, 2007, *Improving Services and Support for Older People with Mental Health Problems*, London: Age Concern.

Waugh, E., 1953, 'Frankly speaking', BBC Home Service interview, The Spoken Word, British Library.

5 Building and supporting a partnership

Key messages

- Each organisation should keep under review its potential for merging with another organisation, or entering a consortium or 'sharing services': an annual option appraisal is sensible
- Networks matter as much as hierarchies and organisations
- Partnerships need to go through set stages of development, each of them completed properly before moving on to the next, if they are to become viable, then sustainable
- Organisational development is a pre-requisite of a successful partnership
- Some partnership programmes have delivered multi-million pounds savings targets through collaborative working
- If there is a single theme to be guided by in building and supporting a partnership, it is: communication, communication, communication

'It's a partnership opportunity'
(Two businessmen overheard on the London underground)

'Toto, I don't believe we are in Kansas anymore'.
(Dorothy, *The Wizard of Oz*)

'Every human benefit, every virtue and every prudent act, is founded on compromise'
(Edmund Burke)

'I am because we are'.
(The collective engagement of peers in South Africa in the process known as Ubuntu)

Types of partnership

Contracts or partnerships?

Social care partnerships take one of three main forms: *contracts, multi-agency partnerships* or *case-specific partnerships.*

Contracts

Contracts set out how a service is to be provided, normally through one agency delivering a commissioned service for another, sometimes based upon a specification the agency or firm will have won competitively, at other times through being granted *preferred partner* status. Contractors should always be seen as partners if they are to take ownership of ownership of the service they are providing, be it an adolescent foster care service, a home care service or a supported housing service. Partnering contracts have replaced adversarial contracts as the industry standard, with a contract now being 'a far more optimistic document, in that it looks forward to what will be achieved in a partnership, providing flexibility for change in a collaborative environment' (Allen 2002). However, all contracts still need to be monitored regularly for compliance.

These days, it is as likely a preferred partner or contractors will have been appointed through either an open, restricted or competitive dialogue, or through a negotiated procedure. Whichever the route, interested applicants are whittled down to a final number through a process of tough questioning about how the applicant will provide the solutions needed by the organisation or body awarding the tender. The 'fit' between a commissioner and contractor, including the ability to work together, is as crucial as the price and volume aspects of a contract. The same shift of emphasis is taking place in adoption assessments, with more emphasis on the 'fit and click' in the matching process between child and potential adopter, as much as a lengthy adoption assessment process conducted without a child in sight.

Multi-agency partnerships

Multi-agency partnerships are formed when a social problem is beyond the ability of any single agency to solve on its own (see Chapter 1). Safeguarding children (previously called child abuse, then child protection) is one such service. A 4-year-old child may need a social worker, a teacher and a health visitor to work together effectively, if that child is to be safeguarded from risks at home. This is an example of a *case-specific partnership* which is replicated at the agency level through a Local Safeguarding Children Board (LSCB), at which all safeguarding agencies like children's services (children's social care services and education services), the police, the health service and probation, are represented. LSCBs meet regularly to establish common procedures, to review cases where children have died or been seriously injured in suspicious circumstances, to improve joint practice and to raise public awareness locally about the grave dangers some children face.

Case-specific partnerships

Most social care cases involve a greater or lesser degree of partnership working. Caring for an older person at home may require several health and social care professionals to work well together, usually a home care worker and a community nurse as a safe minimum. Other specialist staff such as a community pharmacist may also visit as a part of a multi-agency *care plan*. Often, they will record their visits in a diary left in the service user's home, so that each visiting professional can be up to date with what has been done, and with any developments they all need to know. In this way, a *professional network* is established, providing a *personalised service* to a vulnerable adult (or child) living in the community.

Partnerships, or networks, can be short-life or permanent. Many users of social care services need brief, timely help to support them through a crisis. Their crisis might last days, weeks or months. The importance of a small amount of support for an individual or a family should never be under-estimated (see Chapter 1). It often makes the difference between survival or going under. A far smaller group of service users need help for years, decades and, in some cases, life. Whereas a 'life' sentence in penal policy may mean between 10 and 30 years, the life of a social care case can mean literally 'life'.

The answer to the question, *should it be contracts or partnerships*, especially in today's complex and fragmented world, is invariably – both. Most services are likely to be a mixture of contracts and partnerships, with some elements of a contract run more like a partnership, and with even partnerships requiring formal scrutiny.

The networking and negotiating element of contracting is vital to ensure that contracts are let to providers who have a long-term commitment to the awarding body's aims, objectives and values. Similarly, the inter-dependence is such that the awarding body has to be equally committed to understanding the pressures on their contractor or contractors and to be prepared to share risks in a jointly agreed proportion, especially over a long-term contract of 5–10 years, when circumstances will inevitably change beyond recognition.

A merger or something less draconian?

Earlier chapters considered the context for partnership working, and how it is affecting the participants. This chapter considers the agenda for organisations. Joined-up working implies a re-alignment between organisations, and this chapter discusses the various forms this is taking. Options range from closer collaborative arrangements without structural change, through to a full merger.

The main advantage of a merger is to create one set of decision-makers and a single body of intellectual property. Merging is still a significant business strategy, for large and small businesses alike. There were £2.05 trillion worth of merger and acquisition (M&A) deals done in 2006, the most since the M&A boom of 1997–2000. Over the last two years, two French energy giants, Suez and Gaz de France, have merged; West and East Midlands ITV regions are merging to form a single Midlands ITV company; and *Children Now* and *Young Peoples Now* magazine merged, keeping the interest of youth workers by producing monthly supplements on youth work. The UK public sector is big business too. The NHS is the third largest employer in the world after the Chinese army and the Indian railways. Service Birmingham, a joint venture company established by Birmingham City Council and Capita, made £9 million savings in 2007 from their business transformation programme (Marchant 2008).

Over 60 per cent of mergers or change programmes fail for a variety of reasons. A merger being planned between two major voluntary organisations in the UK collapsed because the board of one organisation could not agree to give up what they thought the organisation stood for and represented, despite clear strategic advantages of the proposed merger, which had been planned for over two years.

Where they have the choice, organisations today are tending to opt for collaboration and better co-ordination of what they do, rather than merger or integration, in a 'surge of strategic alliances across the globe' (Sudarsanam 2003). 'Even in a cordial merger, motivation can vaporise overnight', according to Carlos Ghosn, President and CEO of Nissan and Renault. Ghosn's suggestion is to create an 'alliance of equals', rather than acquiring or absorbing companies, because 'companies do not snap together like plastic building blocks' (Ghosn 2006). As Nortel's (the global telecoms group) Chief Strategy Officer, George Riedel says, 'Collaboration involves low to medium organisational inter-dependence, has clear goals on both sides, and a good strategic fit. Although the level of commitment may vary, the terms are inherently flexible. In contrast, mergers eliminate duplication and create a single management team. However they bring challenges associated with cultural fit, revenue slippage, product and technology rationalisation and power struggles' (Riedel 2006). Glisson and Hemmelgarn found that 'efforts to improve children's services should focus on positive organisational climates rather than on increasing inter-organisational services co-ordination' (Glisson and Hemmelgarn 1998).

Aligning without merging has also been described as moving towards increased 'co-opetition' (Bamford *et al.* 2003). In group structures, a number of complementary organisations can join together in a federal arrangement with an overarching board. This is common practice in the social housing sector, enabling a group comprised perhaps of five or six smaller housing associations, to share professional services and absorb financial shifts more easily. Xerox and Fuji Photo Film in Japan have been in a joint venture for over 40 years whilst keeping their separate identities. Speaking of the NHS's penchant for restructuring, the policy analyst Chris Ham suggests that the NHS should be developing integrated clinical networks, rather then encouraging hospitals and trusts to compete with each other over operations and treatments. 'This is OK for younger people facing a simple procedure but not for older patients who have multiple or complex conditions that require treatment by integrated teams of specialists, not treatment of a series of discrete fragmented problems' (Ham 2008).

Mergers and acquisitions are braver, and sometimes the only course of action to take. Many small third-sector organisations will only be able to compete for contracts let by large national or regional commissioners if they merge with one or more organisations to build sufficient capacity to handle large contracts, which may be the only contracts on offer. This has been a constant threat to small voluntary and community organisations, to the point where consideration of a merger strategy should be on the strategic and business plan of every small organisation unless it is confident in its long-term niche market. Livability is a new organisation formed in 2007 through the merger of John Grooms and the Shaftesbury Society, two voluntary organisations caring for disabled people, who as a result of the merger, doubled their capacity and financial base. Other organisations merge in a quest for sector dominance, to avoid the complete financial meltdown of one partner, or to increase their combined geographical spread and ability to influence government policy.

Voluntary sector organisations have always merged, particularly when a larger organisation absorbs a smaller organisation on the point of financial collapse or when it is no longer viable (see 'Reflections on a merger' box). Deals are often sealed at so-called 'amalgamation dinners' between the two respective boards. Vertical integration is also an important means of reducing inconsistency in a national service. That is the reason Victim Support brought 89 of its local independent services into a single national organisation for the first time in 2008. Many proposed mergers come to nothing, because they are a great idea of a powerful individual, but lack a grounding in reality, such as the request in 1956 by Guy Mollet, the anglophile French Prime Minister, that France should become part of England.

Governments and mergers

Governments within the UK have been keen in recent years to promote public sector mergers, in order to rationalise, to unify disparate groups of related services, to promote more joined-up working on behalf of UK citizens, and to deliver efficiency savings. Examples of rationalisations and mergers are:

- The SNP Government's policy of 'de-cluttering' the landscape of civil service quangos, starting with the merger of Scottish Screen and the Scottish Arts Council, and the likely abolition of the housing quango, Communities Scotland.

Reflections on a merger

In 2006, the Family Services Unit (FSU) a charity which had provided support services to hard-to-reach children and families of all descriptions through 59 local services in England and Scotland since 1948, merged in England with the Family Welfare Association, a national charity with a similar mission, and in Scotland with a new independent charity, CIRCLE, which has attracted support from several media and showbiz people and through them, a new funding base.

Six ex-FSU regional managers and many front-line staff, based in London, Leicester, Birmingham, Manchester, Sheffield and Bradford, now work for FWA. The view of FSU staff is that the merger was successful because the FSU legacy and its distinctive contribution to social work with families has been kept alive within FWA. There is a broad consensus that non-statutory preventative work shrank hugely in the 1990's and it is good to have some surviving practitioners.

FWA welcomed FSU, its staff and its values, initially as outsiders within, with a view to growing shared values over time. FWA's positive approach and openness at a time when FSU would have soon ceased to exist due to declining income and rising pension liabilities, is a lesson for other charities faced with the 'vulnerability of smallness' or another compelling driver to merge, about the type of organisation they might wish to approach.

- In England, all NHS Trusts had to apply for Foundation Trust or Social Enterprise status by April 2008. This had the disadvantage of constant structural change, with the risks of distraction, although it also offered opportunities.
- Oxfordshire Learning Disability NHS Trust applied to become a social firm/social enterprise, in order to meet the needs of people who use its services more flexibly outside of the NHS structure and culture.
- HMRC was created out of the Inland Revenue and Customs and Excise in 2005 and the UK Borders Agency, from the merger of the Customs, Border and Immigration Agency and UK Visas service, in 2008.
- Nine new unitary councils will be formed in 2009 in England, causing a major re-alignment for the counties who previously provided their own direct services.
- Many councils are combining in whole or in part, sometimes with other public sector agencies, especially local primary care trusts. These moves are part of a trend towards co-government (see below).

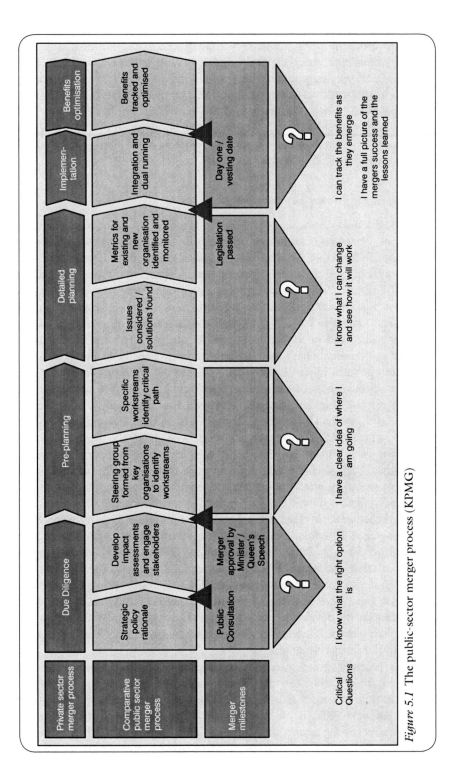

Figure 5.1 The public-sector merger process (KPMG)

Co-government in the public sector mirrors large international consortia in the private sector, especially in the delivery of intergovernmental contracts. The A380, the largest plane in the world, with 300 miles of wiring in each plane, is made by Airbus as a single integrated company, absorbing businesses from the UK, France, Germany and Spain. Wings are made in the UK, and the fuselage and cabin in Germany. Questions remain about whether this degree of integration is efficient, or whether it leads to a fragmented structure with insufficiently clear authority.

Public/private finance partnerships

In 1998, Frank Dobson, the then Health Secretary, published a consultation document, *Partnership in Action*, in which he famously advocated bringing down the 'Berlin Wall' between health and social services. The same could be said for bringing down the financial wall between the public and private sectors. Until the 1980s, social care was a near-monopoly state service, apart from the use of unregulated private care homes for vulnerable children and adults. Over the last 20 years, as a direct result of government policy on 'best value' and on reducing the public sector borrowing requirement (PSBR), governments have encouraged the private sector to invest in social care developments, in a mixed economy of care model of public, private and voluntary providers, and through establishing joint venture companies or 'special purpose vehicles', like that between the East Riding of Yorkshire Council and Arvato Government Services Ltd. Other examples are private finance initiative (PFI) schemes, in services such as the re-provision of residential care homes into smaller 'homelier' and often dual-registered care homes (suitable for residential and nursing home care), so that, once admitted, a resident would never need to move again however frail or unwell she or he might become.

Many schemes are in place, and are now in the middle of long-term contracts and repayment schedules, impacting on commissioning organisations like a mortgage debt. By 2007, the Department of Health had invested £438 million in adult social care PFI Schemes in England, with the Department of Communities and Local Government (DCLG) contributing £83 million. Critics say the PFI debt is too large and the interest payments unjustifiable. Supporters say the developments would never have been built without private finance taking the risk, especially given restrictions on council's ability to raise capital in the financial markets.

More recently, governments have sought or stipulated more national co-ordination of public/private finance initiatives, to minimise the risk of fragmentation amongst individual franchisees, contractors and suppliers. British Railways (BR) is an example, as it has fragmented into Network Rail and a revolving group of train companies, compared with the French equivalent, SNCF, 170 years old and still a single integrated national service, and having orchestrated the sort of punctual high-speed rail network Britain can only dream about.

Lessons are being learnt. For example, the Strategic Investment Board in Northern Ireland was set up in 2003 to co-ordinate all public infrastructure programmes. 'Rather than starting from the separate demands of Northern Ireland's 11 government departments, the Board has identified six overarching areas: networks, skills, health, social, environment and productive' (*Financial Times*, 17 January 2008). The trend towards governments retaining control in order to co-ordinate strategic developments shows the limitation of the private sector taking over key areas of a government's statutory responsibility, and how reckless it can be to devolve accountability or the levers of power.

Partnerships through a consortium or consortia

Consortia are big business too. In 2006, a consortium of 157 NHS trusts pooled their IT purchase volumes and participated in an online 'reverse' auction, with suppliers bidding lower prices against each other to establish the lowest possible price. The negotiation between trusts sought to build a commercially viable consensus.

A consortium is a voluntary agreement between agencies to act together to commission or provide a service. The most common consortia in the UK are collaborative commissioning consortia, adoption consortia and consortia to provide support to asylum seekers. Through a joint commissioning unit, local authorities in Greater Manchester (Bolton, Bury, Manchester, Oldham, Rochdale, Salford, Stockport, Tameside, Trafford and Wigan), through the Association of Greater Manchester Authorities (AGMA), with Blackburn with Darwen, Blackpool and Warrington councils as associate members, form the Greater Manchester Benefits Consortium, claiming multi-million pound savings. The AGMA also jointly commissions out-of-authority placements for children. Similarly, West London Authorities (WLA) claim multi-million pound savings on adult commissioning through managing the market and managing annual uplifts claimed by providers down to manageable levels. Six councils in southwest London (Croydon, Merton, Kingston, Richmond, Sutton and Wandsworth) are collaborating to make savings on learning disability services, and to re-shape those services. Gloucestershire County Council has developed a tool for more realistic pricing of high-cost placements across southwest England. It is customary for one agency to be the lead agency for the purpose of hosting a consortium.

An adoption consortium is formed when a number of local authorities or voluntary adoption agencies share details of waiting families and children in order to try to make speedy local placements for children. They may also collaborate in providing post-adoption support and sharing information. Adoption 22 is a consortium of all 22 local authorities in the northwest of England. The South West Adoption Consortium consists of 15 local authorities and three voluntary adoption agencies (VAAs) and the West of

Scotland Family Placement Consortium has 12 local authority members and one VAA.

All UK regions have a consortium to support asylum seekers, either called a regional asylum seekers consortium or a strategic migration partnership. Such steps towards integration are being matched in central government with the establishment of one government department – the Home Office through the Borders Agency – assuming responsibility for funding support for unaccompanied asylum seeking children before and after they turn 18.

Mutual assistance models work well and normally individuals and agencies respond positively to cries for help in exceptional circumstances or in a crisis. It can be harder to mobilise help in quieter times.

Consortia or alliances of organisations in a sector can make it easier to represent the interests of the sector to government, and easier for government to communicate with the sector. This strengthens consensus-building and confidence in each other, and reduces the perception of divide and rule (attributed by a sector to government's motives) and fragmentation and disunity (attributed by government to a sector).

Networks

In partnership working terms, networks are groups of professionals or people who use services who get together, regularly or less frequently, to pursue a common interest. Networks can operate within organisations or across organisations, and can be local, regional national or global. Hosted networks are often called managed networks, as it is a skill to bring together and keep together a group of professionals across geographical and organisational boundaries: network managers are sometimes employed to do this. Women's Aid brings together children's workers from over 60 women's refuges across England for regular support. The Parental Mental Health and Child Welfare Network (www.pmhcwn.org.uk), is hosted by the Social Perspectives Network/Foundation, itself hosted by the Social Care Institute for Excellence (SCIE). Most current service reviews contain a recommendation about establishing a network – 'building a cross-governmental network of shared services professionals, enabling beneficial relationships to be established across a wide range of departments' (National Audit Office 2007).

Communities of practice are self-organising networks of practitioners interested in a particular aspect of practice (Wenger 1998). Other networks include short-life networks, set up to organise action in response to a particular event, and teams around service users – the 'team around the child' model of care, which defines the roles of different professionals working together with a lead professional ensuring care is provided coherently (see Kurrajong Early Intervention Service (www.kurrajongwaratah.org.au); and the 'team around the practitioner', assembled to give maximum support to a practitioner under threat or stress or who perhaps needs radical learning measures.

Care has to be taken not to let the team around the child (or practitioner) become the crowd around the child (or practitioner), which is a risk when so many new professional roles have been established in a short period of time. For example, Connexions was set up in 2001 to be a one-stop advice service for 13–19-year-olds, but by 2008, young people almost need an advisor to work out which advisor they need, given the rise in the numbers and types of mentors for specific issues. Some leaders and managers now argue that it is more realistic to think of organisations as networks rather than hierarchies, including the NHS, which has its own Partners Network to promote good joint working and information sharing about best practice.

Networking has parallels in all aspects of social care practice, including business processes. Construction design management (CDM) is a procurement route based upon a problem-solving project management culture, emphasising the 'cultivation of direct long-term relationships with trade contractors … and the importance of co-ordination and management at interfaces between different trade packages' (Langdon and Rawlinson 2006). The construction manager is the network manager, and the team ethos seeks to minimise confrontations between professional teams.

Some networks have a quasi-statutory role, but without teeth. The Family Justice Council is an example, although like many advisory or umbrella groups in different sectors, it develops joint policy positions and produces influential papers on behalf of its sector or industry. Combined strategies or policies are another increasing trend, emerging from networks and alliances.

The importance of networking has been described throughout this book. Another illustration is that when researching what led young British muslims to become suicide bombers in their own country, Shiv Malik found that what mattered was not what people were doing in the months and years before they struck, but who they were associating with, or 'conspiring' with – their networks, not just their actions at the time (Malik 2007).

Co-government

Co-government, originally a term coined in South American radical politics during the 1950s, is an increasing feature of the partnership landscape in the UK. It literally means joint government (Clarke 1998). Examples are where a chief executive runs two councils at the same time, to promote synergy and to make savings, employing dual or triple key arrangements – to guard against any conflict of interest: or where a council and a PCT, as in Herefordshire, decide to merge and form a public service trust, even though this was subsequently not pursued due to being potentially *ultra vires*; or in the new unitary authorities in England such as the Cornwall Unitary Council in which all tiers of government are coming together into a single authority responsible for all local government services. Appointing a service user and senior manager as joint chair of a Partnership Board is another form of co-government, even though the power relationship is imbalanced, and the power of one partner relies totally on influence, not statutory authority. For example, a large local authority with a budget of half a billion pounds, has more power, resources and capacity, than a small local voluntary organisation with a budget of under £10,000, yet the culture between them has to be based on the principle of equal status. Co-government, or power sharing, can be seen increasingly in political coalitions around the world, and is always an option when thinking about how best to develop an equal status partnership. The more radical potential forms of co-government are yet to be developed, between wildly different organisations with a common purpose.

Shared services

One form of co-government is where a service or a small group of services are shared between two or more organisations, in order to provide a greater critical mass of professional skills than is possible in one organisation alone, and to make savings. The Anglia Revenues Partnership (ARP) between Breckland, Forest Heath, and East Cambridgeshire councils delivers a common revenues and benefits service. It is now diversifying to carry out consultancy work to other councils and organisations. The Department for Communities and Local Government (DCLG) sponsored Regional Centre of Excellence, itself being revamped, re-launched and morphed into a new Regional Improvement and Efficiency Partnership, is helping to extend ARP into a large-scale revenues and benefits service covering 46 councils. One authority could administer housing benefits for all, while another administers council tax collection for all, for example.

Nearly all major public sector organisations have developed their own internal shared business services, like the Prison Service Shared Service and NHS Shared Business Services (National Audit Office 2007).

South Oxfordshire DC and Vale of White Horse DC began sharing financial services in 2006. The councils decided they should have an equal allocation of staff to avoid perception of a takeover. Their contract covers revenues, benefits, accountancy, internal audit and benefit fraud prevention. Darlington BC and Stockton-on-Tees BC agreed to collaborate in HR, finance, design and print services, and ICT, and decided not to appoint an external partner or contractor – instead forming a joint in-house partnership. Wyre BC and Fylde BC have many joint services – Wyre provides Fylde's coastal defence and property management services, and both councils have a three-way joint health and safety service with Blackpool council. Many councils share individual posts such as joint procurement officers. Essex has a procurement 'hub' with a joint team covering seven councils, and Suffolk County Council hosts a virtual legal services team across the county council and seven district councils, where any member of any legal team can ring the strongest point of expertise within the combined virtual team.

Before entering a shared services agreement, it is essential that organisations are transparent about their own costs, especially for those corporate services

Surrey Shared Services: 'you can't buy a goat from us to keep your meadows down'

The quote refers to one of the many questions answered by the call centre of Surrey County Council's shared services team. The service was developed as a joint venture with IBM though the council is taking back an increasing number of functions from IBM by Year 4 of a 10-year contract, a common trend in such joint ventures. The service has expanded to now hold 47 payroll contracts, including all schools in Surrey and the county's probation service. The shared services centre was set up in nine months, comprising an information bureau and back-office teams. Major savings in administration were made, including halving the numbers of staff needed to carry out the same functions previously undertaken in separate departments, without the need for compulsory redundancies. The service is run on a total efficiency model with personal relationships between staff in shared services and departments being deliberately broken down, emphasising the transactional relationship. The biggest culture shift for the whole organisation was to move from paper to electronic forms, and to require staff to adopt a self-service model for most day-to-day transactions.

In common with findings from other shared service arrangements, the centre's work has led to faster and more robust transaction processing, and better management information.

Source: Debra Maxwell, Head of Shared Services,
Surrey County Council

most likely to be shared, as 'there is a lack of transparent data about the costs of public bodies' existing corporate services' (National Audit Office 2007). The NAO also found that, despite best practice examples like those described above, 'there has been little focus on measuring the performance of corporate services and demonstrating how it can be improved through shared services' and 'while shared services are on course to deliver financial savings, current levels of customer satisfaction do not yet present a compelling case for others to follow the same route' (National Audit Office 2007).

Multi-agency teams

The last two decades have witnessed the rise and rise of multi-agency teams, to the point where nearly all social care services are now organised through them. Teams vary in size and role division but very few single agency teams remain in place, and where they do, they risk structural isolation from other agencies operating in their field.

Early joint teams like community mental health teams, youth offending teams and community learning disability teams have acted as role models for new multi-agency teams, including children looked after teams, who mostly now have a health visitor, a nurse and perhaps a teacher as core members of the team, children's cancer support teams, and children's rheumatology teams.

The growth rate in new multi-agency teams is staggering. Many councils like Shropshire, and Telford and Wrekin, have recently restructured into new multi-agency teams for integrated service delivery, producing higher contact rates with new mothers in Telford as one immediate outcome. In Sedgefield, County Durham, adult social care, housing and health services are being reorganised into five neighbourhood level multi-disciplinary teams (district nurses, social workers and housing support officers). Whilst GPs in Sedgefield lost nurses to these teams, they gained more social work and housing support. Essex proposed between 25 and 30 local multi-disciplinary teams (TASCCs – teams around schools, children and communities) with a strong focus on early intervention and prevention – 'The Council's ambition is to make a difference to all children. Evidence from our Braintree Pathfinder Children's Trust and from numerous other pilots around the county, is that by extending our range of activities into preventive and early intervention work and by working more closely with services such as schools and health that exist for all children, we can make more difference and offset some of the demand for more complex responses' (Essex County Council Cabinet report 2006). By 2008, there will be a further 49 children's centres in Essex, which offer potential bases for new teams, though concerns were being expressed that the proper focus on safeguarding was becoming diluted

Some multi-agency team developments bring positive service developments and risks at the same time and in equal measure.

A joint benefits assessment service between Sutton Council and the Department for Work and Pensions (DWP), created a home-based one-stop shop for benefit assessments from different public-sector bodies. A joint accreditation process enables staff from the respective agencies to carry out each other's financial assessments. However, concerns about such joint financial assessment teams are strong, especially amongst some welfare rights advisors who worry that the joint team only targets a small number of pensioners receiving care – only 4 per cent of people over 60 receive a social care service, and that this is merely a referral protocol, not a joint team. Better practice, they argue, is joint take-up campaigns built up between welfare rights services and the local DWP service. The DWP programme means independent advocacy agencies are having their funding scaled back because their local authority has a joint team. Local authority welfare rights staff feel their advocacy role on benefits is being constrained, and voluntary organisations feel that they are having to become involved in assessing claimants for non-compliance, a parallel disillusionment to that taking place in the Probation Service with the policy emphasis on enforcement, not rehabilitation. It is important to carry out an impact assessment of how a new joint service impacts upon the morale and motivation of practitioners.

Preparing for partnership development

Classifying the stages of partnership development

Partnerships are classified by type, process and chronology, in a 'proliferation of taxonomies' (Peck and Crawford 2004). Here are some examples.

Frost's classification of the types of partnership has four levels, with co-operation as Level 1, collaboration as Level 2, co-ordination as Level 3 and merger/integration as Level 4 (Frost 2005).

Hudson *et al.* (1999) described partnership development as a continuum from isolation to encounter, communication, collaboration and, finally, integration: Elbeik and Thomas as a six-stage process based on defining, planning, team building, control, communications and review/exit (Elbeik and Thomas 1998).

Leutz proposed six laws of integration (Leutz 1999):

1   You can integrate some of the services all of the time, all of the services some of the time, but you can't integrate all of the services all of the time.
2   Integration costs before it pays.
3   Your integration is my fragmentation.
4   You can't integrate a square peg and a round hole.
5   S/he who integrates calls the tune.
6   All integration is local.

O'Cinneide and Keane (1990) set out the following sequence:

1   Preparation of an agreed framework as to how the planning is to be undertaken.
2   A SWOT (strengths, weaknesses, opportunities and threats) analysis.
3   Assessment of what types of interventions already exist, and where the gaps are.
4   Preparation of alternative scenarios.
5   Selection of preferred scenario and prioritisation of actions.
6   On-going monitoring and periodic evaluations.

The Institute for Voluntary Action Research (IVAR) advises organisations about four discrete stages: negotiation: decision-taking: planning; and implementation (IVAR 2008).

More romantically, Taylor *et al.* (2003), classified partnership development in terms of the first date – developing the relationship, tying the knot, keeping going and moving on, also a 'co-evolution of culture and structure, each shaping and in turn being shaped by the other' (Bate *et al.* 2000). Such co-evolution is likely to be permanently ambiguous, and attempts to resolve it are often counter-productive. Healthy co-existence is often more comfortable and therefore more productive for participants.

Gloucestershire County Council, in collaboration with the Tavistock Institute, reviewed their strategic partnerships and developed a cycle of partnership based upon 'deliberation, authorisation, implementation and evaluation' (Swann 2007).

Each of these classifications has merit and can be used, or all of them can be used to refer to as, despite their differences, they are essentially descriptors of a process which can be divided into the same clearly defined stages (see below).

Project management

Whichever, if any, classification is adopted, all partnerships need to be developed through a clear project management framework. They need to be well planned, well run, well co-ordinated, regularly reviewed and well delivered (see box for an example from the management of a project to group all town hall services, delivered from separate buildings around a town, onto a single site in a new town hall). Various methodologies can help to structure projects, such as Prince 2. The most crucial role is that of the project manager. His or her role is to co-ordinate different workstreams and deliver the overall project. As Fletcher says, 'the competence of the project manager is critical to the success of the project. A good project manager has two key characteristics: she is a good people manager, leader and motivator; and a highly systematic, almost obsessional, process manager' (Fletcher 2006).

There are now over 500 professional project directors working in the public sector with experience of completing major projects, using best practice frameworks like *Managing Successful Programmes (MSP)*, and other programmes validated by the Office for Government Commerce (OGC at www.ogc.gov.uk). Whilst this is a strong professional base, more training for project managers is needed (National Audit Office 2008). Project management can be supported by management theories which have a track record of being successfully applied like the Toyota Production System (TPS) (Liker 2004), and Lean Six Sigma (George 2002).

The five stages of partnership development

Stage 1: The big idea

Most partnerships start with a big idea, so the question 'what's the big idea?' is relevant! The best organisations create an environment in which big ideas can be expressed and nurtured.

Town Hall Delivery Project: snapshot of progress

Programme planning and progress: **G**	Next steps: • Gain agreement to Programme Governance proposals • Establish Programme Boards as necessary • Finalise and agree Programme Definition Documents • Further develop milestone plans, project structures and reporting processes • Establish further programme resources • Finalise building purchase • Agree and begin implementation of enhancement works to new building • Continue service consolidation in old campus • Plan children's services consolidation proposals • Top down and bottom up research for area office programme
Programme issues and risks: **A**	Risks: • Length of time to complete new build purchase causes delay to fit-out and therefore the occupation milestones • Data Centre scope for new building potentially far exceeds original expected requirement which could mean significant implications on the Mechanical & Electrical installation and therefore cost and time – clarification on data centre scope being sought
Programme costs: **G**	Costs: • Budget costs being developed as programme definitions become clearer

G (green): on track
A (amber): on track but some caution being expressed
R (red): not on track

Logical framework analysis (log frames) is a means of bringing partners together to plan for the future, particularly to identify their key goals, say in five or ten years' time, and then to look at the steps that have to be taken each year to deliver those long-term objectives. Search conferences fulfil a similar function, by bringing all those with a stake in the future of a service together to brainstorm the best way forward.

The Home Office and PriceWaterhouseCoopers identified the potential for £250 million savings on prisoner movements, through detailed frontline process change, and by a significant increase in the use of video links from prisons to courts. That is an example of a partnership project with a clear purpose and with something of value to pursue for all stakeholders – except perhaps prisoners themselves!

Pre-conditions for partnership working

Partnerships only work if certain pre-conditions are met. Without these pre-conditions, a partnership will be like an aircraft trying to take off with insufficient fuel, without a pilot, without a technical support team, or without a sufficiently long runway to take off from in the first place – it just won't fly. Creating the right conditions for partnership working is a subtle art. Partners should always be chosen carefully. A key question for one organisation to ask itself about another is, 'what is this organisation we're proposing to partner with really like?' After all, you wouldn't buy a house without carrying out a survey. As Sull comments, 'managers can improve the odds of a smooth relationship by screening potential partners for compatibility' (Sull 2001). Similarly, Atkinson *et al.* (2002) emphasise that the 'commitment to and a willingness to be involved in multi-agency working, whatever the type, was felt to be the key to effective collaboration. What emerged was the importance of those involved wanting to be involved and having a belief in multi-agency working, rather than being directed to engage in it'. These attitudes help to create the environment in which a bid idea can be generated, heard and acted upon, adding up to an overall 'readiness to proceed'.

Stage 2: The feasibility study

A good question to ask when thinking about partnership working is 'why change at all?' if the risks are so great. As Drexler said about applying nanotechnology, 'There are many people, including myself, who are quite queasy about the consequences of this technology for the future. We are talking about changing so many things that the risk of society handling it poorly through lack of preparation is very large' (Drexler 1995).

The starting point for partnership working is that existing organisations are probably working as closed systems (Springett 1995). People who use services are viewed from different perspectives, as described in Chapter 3. Accounting systems are different. Decisions are based upon different priority

The dream that got away

The Saxmundham Integrated Health and Social Care Centre, near to the east Suffolk coast, was the dream of Dr John Havard, one of the partners in the town's main GP practice. The centre, to be built on the edge of Saxmundham, had the backing of local statutory partners and included a base for GPs and PCT staff, a pharmacy, accommodation for the local social care team, a day nursery and crèche, an ambulance station, a birthing unit, a training and education centre and a café. Despite some opposition from existing town retailers who felt that the pharmacy would put the town's chemist out of business, the project received a green light from all involved and years were spent securing the commitment of partners and building confidence that the development really would happen.

However, the project collapsed at the eleventh hour due to the local PCT rejecting the business case for the centre, because it needed the money to fund higher priority schemes. The centre had been years in the dreaming, the persuading and the negotiating. The moment, if there ever was one, had passed. With over 1,000 new homes being built in the town, the need for such a centre in this town, as in so many others, was becoming increasingly important. Today, the partners continue as they always have done, seeing patients every day, but with an air of anti-climax and disillusionment.

systems, such as clinical need in the NHS, and on the best interests of children and vulnerable adults in social care. Power and status is also different between partners. In many GP practices, the doctors are partners and employers of other practice staff like nurses, which adds an employer relationship to the pre-existing status gap between doctors and nurses, however positive the level of joint working.

A feasibility study has to analyse the reasons a partnership is likely to fail – eschewing a presumption of success – alongside a hard-headed evaluation of the business case, the capacity to deliver the project and the political ambience surrounding the development.

Amongst innumerable templates for a feasibility study, are force field analysis, mapping exercises, a concept analysis framework (Walker and Avant 1995), proximity exercises, game theory, which suggests that partnerships depend on agencies being in a managed equilibrium with each other (Von Neumann and Morgenstern 1944), or a SWOT (strengths, weaknesses, opportunities and threats) analysis.

Each of them can be useful in helping to set out the key issues that have to be considered, like these below:

- Can the partners demonstrate *mutual gain*? Mutual gain is when each member of a partnership furthers their own separate objectives through being in the partnership. Successful partnerships are selfish, not selfless.
- Does the partnership have *clear objectives*, each of which has a sufficiently high priority for each partner to guarantee their active involvement from the beginning to the end of the partnership?
- Is the partnership *adequately resourced* for the length of time needed to deliver results?
- Does the partnership have *a respected and accepted leader or leaders* who can carry others with them?
- Does the partnership have *the right mix of staff time and abilities* to deliver a complex set of inter-locking tasks?
- Is a formal partnership *a better option* than spending the time co-ordinating services well?

A properly carried out feasibility study, including business cases and risk assessments, will ensure the essential pre-conditions are met. Sound preparation is a major determinant of later success.

Stage 3: Getting started

In starting a partnership project, it is crucial to build a hegemonic group, in Gramsci's terms, who are united, motivated and on board, all setting off at the same time, all going in the same direction and all travelling at the same speed (Jones 2006). Many partnership projects are asynchronous, with nothing on the same timeline, and they will almost certainly fail. It was no coincidence that the first four care trusts in England were located in Health Action Zones, with an immediate pre-history of strong partnership working. (Peck *et al.* 2002). The first children's trust in England to fully integrate children's health services, Brighton and Hove, also had a long history of strong inter-agency working. The industrialist John Harvey-Jones argued for a gatekeeper from each organisation in a partnership to be appointed as a representative or emissary to start to understand the culture of the other partner (private conversation).

It takes nine months to have a baby, no matter how many people you put on the job! Similarly, in the first year of a partnership programme or project, that programme or project needs to pass through set stages. A clear project plan is essential (see Figure 5.2). Early problems are inevitable. It is the same with any new start. One-third of teachers, social workers and nurses decide to leave their profession within the first year, and the 6–9 month point is the point of maximum vulnerability, when the reality of a job starts to sink in, rather than the dreams you start with (Douglas 2002). 'The same is true in business. Companies found they did not start post-deal planning early enough. Although a big difference in organisational culture was the second biggest post-deal challenge, 80 per cent of companies were not well prepared

Action Plan for Anyborough 2008 to 2009

	2008											2009			
	Feb	Mar	Apr	May	Jun	Jul	Aug	Sep	Oct	Nov	Dec	Jan	Feb	Mar	Apr
1) Corporate Management team augmented as appropriate by elected members and health personnel and Older Persons' Advisory Group consider a vision of life in old age to which they are prepared to commit time and resourcing – 1 month			➤												
2) A broader-based visioning event with large representation of older people and front line staff – facilitated by at least two members of group in 1 above – taking place within 2 months of 1 above				★											
3) Senior Member and Officer representatives of City Council and the Health Economy consider what aspects of the recommendation of this review they are prepared to endorse, outline the structural and policy change required – 2 months					➤										
4) Multi-disciplinary Project Team including representatives from Older Persons' Advisory Group and RSLs identified to take forward identification – establish within 2 weeks of 3 above						➤									
5) A subgroup of the Multi-disciplinary Project team augmented as appropriate consider the presentation and resourcing of an extra care village. Detailed costing and site investigations pursued with an objective of bringing forward proposals for funding in 2009–10							➤								
6) Project Team established to work through the details of development of new policy and management and funding of existing extra care (extra care sheltered housing schemes) – with aim to go live in 2008					➤										

Figure 5.2 Anyborough project plan (Source: Care Services Improvement Partnership (CSIP))

Developing a new children's trust through a clearly structured process of management

The arrival of a new Chief Executive for Brighton and Hove Council, David Panter, in 2001, who was previously an NHS Chief Executive committed to partnership working, was a vital early building block in the formation of the Brighton and Hove Children's Trust, perhaps the most well-developed partnership trust to date. David Hawker, then Director of Education, began to take on a wider set of children's services responsibilities. His first appointment, in 2003, was James Dougan as joint health and social care commissioner. Hawker then commissioned a series of Best Value Reviews reporting in 2005 on a wide range of services, including CAMHS, early years and children with disabilities – this review led to the establishment of an integrated child development service. The key strategic decision was to put in place co-located multi-agency teams for every children's service, using an age-group approach. Early years services were led by health visitors; 5–13s services by educational psychologists; and adolescents services by Connexions and local authority social workers. In December 2005, South Downs NHS Community Health Trust agreed to second 250 NHS staff into the fledgling children's trust. The next phase of development work included joint HR procedures, an integrated staff supervision policy, and a unified Serious Case Review (SCR) and Serious Untoward Incident (SUI) policy. In 2006, a Children and Young Peoples Trust Board was formed. By 2008, the trust had become a managed network of 6,000 staff and over 500 organisations.

to handle this. It took on average nine months for companies to feel they had control of the significant issues facing the business post-deal' (KPMG 2006). Building 'foreseeability' into partnership agreements is important. Using a 'Partnership Readiness Framework' can help to clarify whether the 'partnership basics' are in place (Greig and Poxton 2001).

Stage 4: Keeping going – the stamina stage: 'I'm not high-maintenance. The situation is high-maintenance' – a woman I overheard speaking to a man at dinner

In this stage, attention often wonders away from the project. Once the inevitable honeymoon period is inevitably over, the fire needs to be re-kindled – partnerships are high maintenance. Expectations have to be managed. If relationships break down, they have to be repaired. If there is a contractual hitch, and there are usually many, it must be remedied quickly. It helps if a project team stays together throughout the programme. Running partnering workshops throughout the course of a programme can maximise engagement by those who will be working in the joint service (4Ps 2008).

As Jim Collins says:

> In building a great institution there is no single defining action, ... no one killer innovation, no solitary lucky break, no miracle moment. Rather our research showed that it feels like turning a giant, heavy flywheel. Pushing with great effort – days, weeks and months of work, with almost imperceptible progress – you finally get the flywheel to inch forward. ... You keep pushing and with persistent effort you eventually get the flywheel to complete one entire turn. You don't stop. You keep pushing in an intelligent and consistent direction and the flywheel moves a bit faster. You keep pushing and you get two turns ... then four ... then eight ... the flywheel builds momentum ... you keep pushing ... thirty-two ... a hundred ... moving faster with each turn ... a thousand ... ten thousand ... a hundred thousand. Then at some point – breakthrough! Each turn builds upon previous work, compounding your investment of effort. The flywheel flies forward with almost unstoppable momentum. This is how you build greatness.
>
> (Collins 2006)

The Collins quote illustrates the importance of maintaining a clear vision of why the partnership is being developed throughout each of the five stages. The risk that short-term issues become pre-occupying is considerable, but that can mean the focus on why the journey was embarked upon in the first place can easily be lost. Sometimes it is genuinely lost, and participants have moved on in their thinking or other priorities take over, so adapting and modifying a project to deal with current problems and pressures in a 'design and build' approach to partnership development, helps to keep programmes relevant and on track.

Conflict resolution

Conflict is endemic in partnerships, given the various statutory functions, business plans and personalities 'in play' at any one time, even with a common purpose. The ability to manage and resolve conflict is important to build into a successful partnership, using an agreed method (see 'Principles of conflict resolution' box).

Many social care partnership programmes take a generation to fully deliver – they are that complex. People with a learning disability have been moving on from NHS long-stay hospitals for over 25 years, yet at the time of writing (May 2008), at least 1,500 people remain on NHS campuses (Department of Health figures). The programmes have had a huge number of people involved, including several changes of political and professional leadership, but momentum has been maintained by people who use services and campaigning

Principles of conflict resolution (formulated by the Diversity Hub)

1   Underlying incompatible positions are always compatible interests. The goal is to reach underneath the rigid position taken to find them.

2   Every side usually has something correct it is trying to communicate.

3   Develop a dialectic process instead of polarising the issue in such a way that people are forced into taking a rigid position.

4   The best way to open a dialectic process is to create an environment where people can express their feelings and concerns without debate. Listening is not the same as agreeing.

5   Parties will often focus on areas of disagreement, even when there are larger areas of agreement – it is important to remind them of the many broad areas of agreement.

6   Decrease defensiveness. A relaxed confident tone is more likely to decrease defensiveness on either side.

7   Place your agenda on the back burner. Stating 'your' needs should usually only proceed after enough contact and goodwill has been established on the other side.

8   It is more effective to step back and think about what you are trying to achieve, what the other side is trying to achieve, and then work out how to make it easier for the other side to give you what you need.

9   Ensure you create a range of possible ways people can communicate their concerns. A one-size fits all approach to conflict resolution takes no account of diversity and militates against good outcomes.

(The Diversity Hub 2006)

groups on their behalf, including networks of committed learning disability professionals for whom the programme has been an important part of their professional lives – whichever job they are in, the values associated with the programme have remained intact. Value-based interviewing can help to ensure whoever is appointed to key roles within a programme like this, shares the vision so that they can come into the programme already committed (see a fuller description later in this chapter).

Stage 5: Sustainability, or finish and move on

To be sustainable, partnerships must continue to make sense at a number of levels over a period of time which will inevitably include changes in

The universal banking programme: from giros to bank accounts

This programme aimed to move benefit and tax credit customers from being paid by giro, to having money paid into new bank accounts set up for this purpose. The programme also aimed to be a first step toward financial inclusion for people in receipt of giros who had traditionally been refused a bank account. The lead role for the programme sat within the Department for Work and Pensions (DWP), with the main partners being the ten largest banks in the UK, the Post Office, the Department for Trade and Industry (DTI) and the Inland Revenue. The programme leader, Shirley Trundle, called 'the Universal Banking Programme Director', was accountable to a specially established cabinet subcommittee, which reflected the high political priority accorded to the programme. This was much needed as partners had separate agendas and no shared set of interests to begin with, and the programme team had no direct leverage.

The key transformations in the programme were unlocking the previous policy logjam across government about how this should be done, and getting the banks on board – they were reluctantly corralled through being reminded about the corporate social responsibility agenda. The project worked more smoothly at junior levels within partner agencies, where specialists simply got on with it as a relatively straightforward task, unlike many of their superiors who were sometimes attempting to recreate the policy logjam.

Use of giros went down from 58 per cent to under 5 per cent between 2002 and 2006, creating more than £1 billion savings over five years, and enabling some of the poorest people in society to be able to hold a basic, no overdraft bank account, or a new Post Office Card Account.

personnel, objectives and financing. Many major partnerships are now over 20 years old, and have adapted to serial changes in their external environment. Through a partnership between Kent County Council and Rowse and Associates going back to 1988, a new town and community, Kingsmill, was built on the site of the old West Malling airfield in north Kent, in an example of a long-term partnership which is continuing to deliver and exceed its original objectives.

Other major projects can be completed within a shorter time-scale (see 'The universal banking programme' box). Each project is unique and its project plan has to be customised to the *n*th degree.

There are several useful books about successful change management, including an excellent fable about penguins who live on an iceberg that is melting, and how they learn to live without a fixed point of reference (Kotter 2006).

Exit strategies

Endings are no easier than beginnings. In fact there are very few clean endings. Daimler and Chrysler merged in 1998, and in 2007 looked ready to part, either through a total merger or clean break. Chrysler cars have stalled whilst Mercedes continued to grow. Many foreign investors in China have found recently that Chinese firms who started off as their junior partners, are now developing equal global ambitions and are no longer content to play a secondary, dependent role.

When a contract, project or service ends, it is important it ends well, with positive 'closure', as many participants may find themselves working together again with different hats on. It is important blame is avoided if the programme ends prematurely or acrimoniously. Of course blame is often warranted and it is part of being accountable, but it is nearly always best to pursue a 'lessons learned' approach, so that spirit of joint working is maintained rather than it appearing something doomed from the start.

Supporting partnership development

Risk management

On 9/11, as the terrorist pilots approached the twin towers, they turned the throttle on the planes to full speed on impact in order to kill the maximum number of people. Only one of the towers was insured, and whilst the owners claimed that what happened was a single event, insurance companies still only paid out on the one tower. The widespread implications of this unforeseeable event included hitherto unparalleled terrorist behaviour.

Politicians dislike surprises, and being a politician around social care services is high risk, as the nature of the work is steeped as much in failure, disasters and near-misses as successes. A near-miss is often the way social care agencies are alerted to a group of service users they have let down or lost sight of, when they have to urgently instigate reviews and emergency action on cases. Everyone involved in social care, including politicians, needs a healthy 'risk appetite'.

Not all risks can be avoided. There is a 1 in 3,000 risk of radiation damage from a CT brain scan in children, but which parent or paediatrician would not be prepared to take that risk? Many home visits by social care staff contain risks to both staff and service users which if they were all risk assessed according to health and safety legislation and guidance, would never go ahead. Many social care decisions, based upon good risk assessments, contain risks of further harm or damage – there are few risk-free decisions. What is important about partnership working is to share information, share decision-taking and share the risks.

The risk of a near-miss can be minimised by procedures such as the standard clinical triple check before a patient goes into surgery – that it is the right patient, the right operation and the right part of the body. Triple checks are typically undertaken by a consultant, nurse and anaesthetist. In social care, joint working can mean that a second and third opinion on an assessment or judgment are made and recorded, through a multi-disciplinary assessment.

Finance and liability

There are financial and contractual risks in partnership working. The core financials in a partnership may not be understood properly, through an overstatement of the potential benefits. Liability is a key issue in a shared services agreement or partnership. A private-sector company will seek to limit its liability in a shared services arrangement or partnership, seeking to limit recoverable losses by excluding indirect losses, loss of profit as well as including a liability cap, which is usually fixed as a multiple of fees paid. It is essential to be clear about change control in a contract, to allow for changing circumstances, preferably change control with mutually agreed mechanisms and incentivising clauses to keep the contract alive for all parties, plus a liquidated damages clause in case of failure to deliver.

There are good risk management toolkits on the market, including the Fame roadmap process.

Developing a positive partnership culture

When anything as trendy or as obligatory as partnership working assumes 'undeniability status', yet when staff or agencies see no point in it, a syndrome of 'partnership faking' can set in, whereby the semblance of partnership working or a virtual partnership is created merely in order to satisfy an expectant outside world. An 'elite unity' remains in place behind the scenes, maintained by those in power intent on preserving the status quo, some of them highly accomplished individuals who balkanise organisations (Wilson 2005).

Forming a partnership is a precondition of some external funding, leading to the wry observation that 'partnership working consists of the temporary suppression of mutual loathing in the interests of mutual greed', which is an example of 'partnership faking'. However, an inward focus militates against successful partnership working, and is the hardest culture change to make. In a weapons decommissioning process, guns and weapons can be handed over, but changing mindsets is the hardest thing of all. When parents separate or divorce, parents move on in time, but their children are often stuck at the point of separation and often need more help to adjust than they receive (Trinder and Kellett 2007).

In a similar vein, collaborationists go through the motions of conforming to a partnership working requirement, to further self-interest. Analysing collaborationism in France during World War Two, Peschanki suggests:

> the collaborationist could be defined as a French citizen who wanted to do more than simply 'work with' (that is, for) the Germans and who did not hesitate to support and demonstrate the necessity of such a collaboration. Support and demonstration: the collaborationist groups all took on this double duty, of propaganda and emblematic action.
>
> (Peschanki *et al.* 1988)

Resistance to partnership working, both active and passive, is inevitable, despite 'working together' being rational and unarguable. Difficulties between professional groups are a major factor (see Chapter 3). Some organisations are extreme sports in themselves, with whom it is virtually impossible at times to communicate. Other reasons are set out in Chapter 7, which looks at the effectiveness of partnership working.

Values are the glue that holds a team, partnership or agency together. An architect I know approaches each commission in his own mind by saying 'each building will be better than the last'. For social workers, that might be expressed as 'each case will be better than my last'. For managers – my next supervision will be my best yet. These are examples of positive value-driven outlooks, which tend to inspire others.

Values can be performance managed, including partnership values, for example by asking the following questions in interviews for jobs (value-based interviewing), or when selecting partners for a project or a contract, or when appraising staff:

- For staff in a residential care home, ask 'how have you put the following value into practice?' – Residents must be shown respect and dignity at all times. Which partners could you involve in the care of 'your' resident to enhance a sense of respect and dignity?
- For staff in a safeguarding service for vulnerable children or adults, ask 'what steps have you taken to understand in depth what is currently happening to each service user on your caseload? Is she/he frightened? Does she/he feel safe? Which partners could you involve to strengthen the sense of safety she/he feels?'
- For all staff – what is your personal partnership footprint, your partnership promoting behaviours? – Name as many as you can.

The NSPCC ask their staff to demonstrate a range of identified values and behaviour, which include 'working together', as part of an appraisal process linked to their pay and reward strategy. Being explicit about the values and behaviour which staff must work to is a lever to strengthen a partnership working culture.

Growing up: changing values

In the next street to where I grew up stood a residential home for people with learning disabilities, in a London suburb in the 1950s. My school mates and I called the residents, who we rarely saw, spastics. The home was run by the Spastics Society, which did not change its name to Scope until 1994. The residents and staff were forced to stay inside most of the time because of a hostile community attitude, and that in itself represented an unwitting collusion with a regime within the home which knew not to let the outside world in.

Twenty-five years later, in 1983, I was working as a social work manager in a local authority, a few streets away from the biggest Victorian hostel for homeless people in Camberwell, known as the Spike, which had been on the site for 120 years, originally as a workhouse for families, and which would finally close in 1985. Over 1,000 men slept at what by then was called the Camberwell Re-Settlement Unit, run by the Department for Health and Social Security (DHSS). Despite being in a linked function with obvious reasons for joint working, our council had no contact with the 'Spike'.

In 2008, the government called for more joint working in response to a report published by the Cabinet Office, *Think Family*, so that there would be 'no wrong door' – contact with any service should offer an open door to a system of joined-up support e.g., a probation officer or a housing officer identifies the adult language difficulties of a client and refers them to English for speakers of other languages (ESOL) training, and that services working with both adults and children take into account family circumstances and responsibilities, e.g., an alcohol treatment service combines treatment with parenting classes while supervised childcare is provided for the children (Social Exclusion Task Force 2008).

In 50 years, an isolated service, its residents treated like pariahs, one of many 'total institutions' (Goffman 1970), has blossomed into a partnership model where by each office, each school, each care home, each day centre, is a potential open door through which anyone in need can walk and be referred to the right place. Whilst the implementation of this vision is a little while off, the transformation in attitudes is remarkable.

Political and managerial leaders of a partnership have a duty to inspire those who work for them with a vision of a positive partnership culture, particularly using their relational power *with* each other, rather than their power over each other (Chambers 2004). This is important if staff resist new policies like direct payments, or the greater involvement of children or adults in service provision, if only because of the greater time it takes and often the greater bureaucratic burden of running personalised services, where each service to an individual has to be carefully crafted. Practical steps to effect a change in culture can be taken. One local authority, faced with low take-up of direct payments because of low staff engagement with suggesting it to service users, would not allow community care assessors to arrange care following an assessment unless they had ruled out direct payments for a specific reason which they had to enter onto the management information system. The computer screen for arranging care could not be accessed unless the direct payment fields had been filled in. To generate learning in a partnership culture, cognitive and affective learning should be equally targeted.

To be successful, a positive continuous dialogue between leaders may need to be sustained for years, and for it to be seen as part of the role of replacement leaders, so that a commitment to a decade or more of constructive dialogue is made by a group of agencies, which is binding on their successor agencies. That can be set out in a local accord or concordat. An example of this is the Dartmouth Conferences, which were instrumental in keeping lines of communication open between America and the Soviet Union from 1960 until today, with annual conferences and more recently task groups, dedicated to a wider peace process within the overall value of improving US/Soviet relations (Voorhees 2002).

All member agencies within a partnership must have equal status, if the partnership is to make substantial progress. Inclusivity is a key value, along with a model of democratic working. Stakeholder confidence, crucial in successful networks and partnerships, will only come from being treated fairly and inclusively, within a high trust environment. Low-trust networks are corrosive and communication eventually stops, or becomes skewed. A key development task for many partnerships is to move from being low trust at start-up, which is inevitable if unwanted change has been imposed, to high trust over time.

Authority in partnerships is often bestowed on a respected leader, who combines personal and positional authority. Partnership behaviours place a strong emphasis on negotiation, persuasion and influence, not a command and control style which is inappropriate in a partnership, unless perhaps it is a war cabinet, but even then a consensus is preferable. 'The good negotiator aims to send both parties away believing they have achieved the right outcome by their own cleverness' (Grayling 2001). This is partnership intelligence, on a par with emotional intelligence as a core skill in partnership working.

Techniques like appreciative enquiry – a structured approach to answering key questions together – can support the development of partnership intelligence, as can cross-organisational learning sets. Managers from some councils and PCTs use action learning sets to support their partnership development. Bromley Council adopted the police's National Intelligence Model, based on short case histories, to outline what can be achieved through partnership.

The Public Law Outline: an inter-agency implementation programme

The Public Law Outline, known to insiders by its suggestive acronym of the PLO, is the new (from April 2008) structured procedure for progressing local authority applications to a family court in England and Wales, in respect of a child who a local authority feels needs to be in public care. It aims to simplify the stages a case goes through to avoid cases taking longer than necessary when, for children, time is short.

I was the chairperson of the inter-agency implementation group for the PLO, with a steering group made up of a judge nominated by the High Court president, a local authority representative, representatives of the Welsh Assembly Government, the courts service, the Legal Services Commission, and the two English ministries, the Department for Children Schools and Families, and the Ministry of Justice, which also covers Wales. My first task was to secure funding from all partners around the table to allow for the development of training materials and to put on training workshops around the country in the run up to implementation.

This was the first occasion judges had worked with other agencies on an implementation programme of this sort. Previously, implementation had been in parallel and one of many issues to work through was whether the judiciary could be part of an inter-agency management team, given their constitutional independence. The different systems and strategies adopted by governments in England and Wales were also a sensitive issue from time to time. During the run-up to implementation and shortly afterwards, critics of the programme expressed concerns that the new procedure was too daunting for local authorities to use, and would lead to large numbers of children being left in dangerous circumstances in the community, a point local authorities refuted, arguing if there were fewer children coming into the system, it was due to the higher levels of family and community support they were providing.

My role was to ensure the programme was delivered on time, with statutory guidance issued to local authorities, a practice direction issued for judges, and an inter-agency training programme delivered to practitioners from all agencies.

The programme was delivered due to goodwill on all sides and an excellent project manager.

In thinking about partnership development, it is important not to separate this from existing development programmes, but to integrate partnership working into them.

Consultancy support for partnership working

Government departments have sponsored new programmes with implementation support teams and sometimes grants. Programmes in England include Quality Protects (1998–2004); Valuing People (2001– continuing today with *Valuing People Now*, and now integrated with the Care Services Improvement Partnership); and the Integrated Care Network (2003, also becoming part of the Care Services Improvement Partnership from 2005). These programmes continue to be backed by government regional offices.

Public-private finance projects have benefited from advice by the 4Ps – local government's procurement support arm, which has multi-disciplinary teams

---

Standing or falling on trust

The Institute for Voluntary Action Research works with a number of partners such as IdEA, local authorities and charities, encouraging cross-sectoral partnership working.

One of their major research programmes, the Partnership Improvement Programme, sought to establish a new 'model of enquiry' for how new partnerships could best be developed. Their experience has been that many partnerships or mergers have failed due to a lack of strategic alignment, shared vision or through poor inter-personal relations between key players, which can include arguments over naming of the new merged organisation, or who will be chair or chief executive, reflecting a deep underlying ambivalence. Mergers, their Director, Ben Cairns, says, ' stand or fall on trust'.

Mergers are the most significant event in the lifetimes of the organisations and individuals going through the process. IVAR works by bringing the six key people from each organisation together to work out the basis for a consensus, and to advise the organisations whether there is a basis to proceed or whether more work is needed to establish a shared vision and a commitment to capacity-building. This iterative process can be a positive outcome in itself, as it promotes a shared understanding of the 'collaborative advantage' of the partnership (Huxham and Vangen 2005).

What is needed to make a new partnership work, according to Cairns, is a shared vision, a common understanding of future roles, good interpersonal skills and relationships and a sound financial model with all possible costs understood and factored in.

for all sectors. One partnership developed by the 4Ps is with the University College of London (UCL) and Constructing Excellence, the cross-industry body set up to promote best practice in large-scale construction projects, to design and deliver consultancy packages for project managers.

Useful reference material on how to support partnership working can be found on the websites of many organisations referred to throughout this book, including IdEA, through its Partnerships and Places Library (www. idea.gov.uk).

The major consultancy firms charge as much for a day's input on partnership working or organisational change as the entire monthly income of an average-sized village in the third world. Organisations are generally better off developing their own internal consultancy capacity, as all will have change programmes running on one subject or several over the next decade – or use free consultancies, of which there are several, or to club together in a knowledge club of some description with like-minded organisations, concentrating on 'knowledge co-creation' (Martin 2006).

More recently, the preferred consulting model or industry standard has shifted towards ' active consulting' – doing it, not just advising how to do it. National Leaders of Education (NLE), supported by the National College for School Leadership (NCSL), have pioneered this approach. Bob Hudson, an acknowledged expert in partnership working, not only evaluated Sedgefield's locality-based multi-agency teams, but helped to 'shape' events, rather than just 'report' on them (Hudson 2006).

The two sisters

Julie Thornton and Jana Veryard are co-trainers and also sisters. They run sessions on how to develop collaborative values within or across organisations. Theirs is a partnership based on growing up together and knowing each other inside-out, despite being temperamental opposites and despite not being on speaking terms for five years when one was pre-adolescent and the other in her mid-teens. Their partnership shows that close personal relationships between co-workers can be of great benefit in running social care programmes, despite the unease this sometimes causes amongst those around them. The behaviours that come with deep personal relationships such as an ease around each other, knowing and sensing each other's cues, and sharing long-term values, offer those being trained a sense of real teamwork to draw upon.

Partnership funding

Cost–benefit analysis

The costs of a social care problem are rarely confined to one agency. The economic burden of mental illness has been estimated at £4.6 billion, made up of the cost of lost employment (£1.7 billion); social security payments (£1.1 billion); NHS costs (£0.59 billion); informal care (£0.4 billion); and local authority social care (£0.25 billion) (Comprehensive Spending Review backing documents, Treasury, 2007). Cash-strapped statutory organisations could release funding through partnership working. Fees for children with special educational needs have risen by 79 per cent in the last six years, and now average £57,000 a year per child. The Audit Commission reported that local authorities had not sat down and worked out what they were spending, leading to 'poor liaison between education, social care and health departments. Children with high support needs will tend to be seen by all three services and there was surprisingly little sharing of information' (Audit Commission 2007).

Whilst a conventional cost–benefit analysis cannot be carried out for partnerships, as some costs are quantifiable and other costs are strategic, Glendinning *et al.* (2000) identified savings to health services through direct payments, as people used their personal assistants to carry out several health-related tasks, and this is one of many examples where a pooled budget could release savings for re-investment on jointly agreed priorities. Some statutory agencies are reluctant to commit funding to a partnership because they want to retain control of their entire budget in case they need to use an underspend on one service to bail out an overspend in another, and do not wish to see any of their budget tied up as it reduces their flexibility. Commissioners also wish to retain the option of commissioning differently in future years, without some of their budget being tied to an existing service or an existing service provider. A balance has to be struck, otherwise providers will not have sufficient time or security remaining on the contract to invest in it.

Not everything costs money. As a challenge to local professionals who they felt were always whingeing about not having the resources to meet expectations, a group of service users with learning disabilities drew up a list of behaviours, or as they called them, a Sale of Opportunities, to show what could be provided without any money whatsoever (see box).

In high-trust partnerships, senior managers in a two organisation partnership or trust tend not to worry excessively about which of each other's costs they may be inadvertently paying. They assume that this will even itself out over time, even though clear audit trails are required to ensure that all everything spent by an agency is in line with what it is legally able to spend it on, and accounts are audited every year by independent auditors. Low-trust partnerships are beset by rumblings and allegations about cost shunting and duplicity. In 2007, Brent Council threatened to take Brent Primary Care

'Sale of opportunities'

- How much does it cost to smile?
- How much does it cost to listen?
- How much does it cost to treat others with respect?
- How much does it cost to set the default on your computer to pt16 or 18 and to use Arial font?
- How much does it cost to talk to us first before you talk to our parents and carers?
- How much does it cost to believe people and take what they say seriously?
- How much does it cost to ask people who they want at their review meetings?
- How much does it cost to leave your bad mood at home?
- How much does it cost to treat us as adults?
- How much does it cost to say you are sorry when you have made a mistake?

Answer –Nothing!

(With thanks to Patti Seward of Suffolk Social Care Services)

Trust (PCT) to court over what it claimed was cost shunting of more than £10 million, in relation to the continuing care costs of NHS long-stay hospital patients now living in the community. Many partnerships fail because one partner believes the other is empire building, asset stripping, or concealing its true financial position.

An independent report commissioned by NHS London cited weak financial management, a divided senior executive team and weak scrutiny by the Brent PCT Board as the main problems (Taylor 2008). Yet even in the most intense conflicts, organisations must continue working together, and, despite the conflicts, Brent Council and PCT – through their Health and Social Care Partnership Board – delivered other programmes like a roll out of new children's centres.

With the worsening NHS financial crisis in 2006/07, other PCTs such as Wiltshire and Hampshire withdrew funding from partnership agreements with local councils for the joint commissioning and provision of community care services, leaving local councils in those areas to foot the bill or cut the service. The PCT network simultaneously claimed that a survey of 59 PCTs showed that tighter eligibility criteria set by adult social care departments had led to cost shunting the other way. Cross-charging is rarely definitive, as it can lead to even more expensive secondary legislation defending a claim, or tit for tat manoeuvres.

Counting the true cost of partnership working

The biggest resource in social care is professional time. Investing in new partnerships, including bidding processes for increased funding, is time-consuming, especially for small charities. The biggest cost is staff time. New developments can lead to massive overheads for little gain and there is a risk that 'the baroque complexity of funding arrangements is damaging the work of many charities' (Cavanagh, 2007). Alignment between Government Departments over funding regimes and formulae needs strengthening.

Effort/efficiency ratios can be low in a partnership, because of the 'let's have another meeting' syndrome – endless time spent in meetings without being able to come to a decision, often because of a lack of project support to carry out tasks in between meetings. Meetings have assumed iconic status in modern management and are generally far too static a mechanism for efficient working. A meeting was originally a sit down break in a procession by Frankish bishops first recorded in 966. We have turned a short break into a bureaucratic art form, though some meetings are necessary and not all can be limited to the ten minutes suggested by Mark McCormack (McCormack 1994), or held standing up as some Japanese companies insist on. These days, in their meetings with the Queen, Privy Councillors always stand as the Queen does not want the meeting to last for long! The opportunity costs of meetings, events and travel costs are rarely factored into calculations of efficiency and productivity. They should always be.

Some financial disincentives to partnership working remain in place. In some schools, head teachers need to keep pupils in their school to retain the funding that goes with them, even if some pupils would be better off in another school. Under European Union procurement rules, some government bodies that buy services rather than provide them in-house incur VAT, which limits the financial attractiveness of shared services agreements. The NHS and local councils have different VAT rules, requiring expensive specialist tax and legal advice before entering a joint arrangement.

Workforce development

Staff engagement

> 'Whatever the problem, the workforce is the solution'.
> Jane Haywood, CEO, CWDC (in private correspondence)

Whatever the role an employee has in a partnership development, she or he will need to share the vision for the partnership, if her or his contribution is to be maximised. Trade unions also need to buy into the vision for them to be able to endorse and recommend it to their members. As Luckhurst suggests, 'it is vital to have a shared vision in which the issues of cost and competitiveness are understood by the trade unions, and employers recognise that the creation of high quality work requires high quality employment' (IPA and Unions 21 2005). A Cabinet Office study found that a shared understanding of the case for reform is more powerful than an 'agenda of concessions' or a formal partnership agreement that simply outlines rights and responsibilities (Cabinet Office 2004).

Pro-actively engaging trade unions and professional associations is important. Unions have a seat on the board of the Sheffield Care Trust and this helps the unions to brief their members, field queries and support the employer's agenda where possible, far more than results from leaving the unions and professional associations on the outside. Some trade unions have positively welcomed partnership developments as they have helped them further their own agenda. 'Many of the branches featured in the report had been able to deal very positively with the challenges posed by integrated provision and grow their membership ... the implementation of new policies had given the union a focus' (Unison 2007). With an increasing number of integrated service roles, and with an increasing number of job descriptions in social care stating that partnership working is a core competence, the need for partnership working between employers, trade unions and professional associations is greater than ever before. Joint working responsibilities need to be written clearly into job descriptions, with clarity about what is expected, especially in a new role. Partnership working between management and trade unions can also allow employers to achieve what they want to, whilst providing reasonable levels of protection for valuable front-line staff, against redundancy for example (IPA 2001).

Workforce development, including harmonising terms and conditions, is a major issue to resolve in partnership working, because 'joint work may be more difficult where there are perceived status differentials between team members' (Hudson 2006). Issues about secondments or a complete staff transfer from one organisation to another under TUPE – or Attached Status in Scotland – need to be worked through. The Cabinet Office statement of Practice on Staff Transfers in the public sector 'COSOP' January 2000, consolidated into the Code of Practice on Workforce Matters in public sector contracts 2005, made it clear that TUPE would apply to staff transfers into new organisations like care trusts unless genuine exceptional reasons applied in a specific situation. However, applying the policy in practice may be judged unaffordable in relation to some developments, and many business cases do not factor in sufficiently pension and redundancy costs, which can be considerable. It is important to create opportunities for displaced staff, especially across organisations, and when thinking of redundancy costs, to think of using that funding to promote staff development instead. Skilled HR support is needed throughout the process.

Leadership

Good leadership and management in partnerships is lateral rather than institutional, leading a diverse workforce rather than a single group. Some headteachers are now leaders of a multi-agency school or a federated school (National College for School Leadership 2007). Leadership of a partnership means being a leader of leaders, possessing convenor legitimacy (McCann and Gray 1986). It also means drawing out the leadership potential of every single member of staff across a partnership – to be leaders in relation to their own professional task. Distributed leadership is a key leadership style in partnerships, to 'enable people throughout the organisation(s) to respond rapidly to change', by empowering them to exercise personal leadership in situations and use their own authority responsibly (Reeves *et al.* 2008). Problems between leaders can be resolved through a 'lock-in' group where leaders literally lock themselves in and bang their own heads together until they find a way forward, in meetings without minutes – what goes on tour, stays on tour.

Credibility also comes from having done the job rather than being shipped in from outside with general management skills. Those days are mostly over. Nowadays you tend to find the railways run by railway specialists, large retail groups by retail specialists, and social care services run by those with experience of managing services for either children or adults, depending on the partnership focus.

For leaders of organisations, it is essential to be aware that no two organisations are the same. Many leaders, successful in one job, fail in their next job, through reproducing the methods that were successful in the first job, without making any allowance for the new context.

As with other selection processes referred to in earlier chapters, a matching process is essential when appointing to a leadership role. As Sir Ronnie Flanagan concluded in his major review of policing in the community and inter-agency context, 'Senior leaders from all agencies should choose the most appropriate individual to lead a partnership irrespective of their organisation' (Flanagan 2008).

Many new leadership roles for partnerships come with an ambiguous set of powers (see Chapter 1), and sometimes with confused accountability. The primary skills needed for these leaders are the ability to influence, persuade, negotiate and problem solve. In many ways, these are the skills needed to run organisations even if you do have total unambiguous control and power. Command and control tomes like *The Grey Book*, which told managers in the NHS in the 1970s exactly what to do down to the last detail, would not work in today's organisations. I recall one of the first senior managers I spoke to in depth about management, in 1983, expressing exasperation with his staff for not carrying out his instructions. His pet phrase, trotted out in a defeatist tone, was 'why won't they just do what they're told?'. He sensed he had lost control, but did not know how to recover: and knowing how to recover from adversity is an essential part of the modern manager's toolkit. Managers also have to be more generous to their staff than their staff may be to them. Leaders and managers are sometimes criticised for being two-faced, but to do their job well they have to be three-faced: facing inwards to staff they directly manage; facing inwardly and outwardly to other professionals and organisations; and facing outside to people who use services.

The role description for a head of a joint team or service can usefully include the following clauses:

- Sees every professional in the joint team as equally important, and translates that value into action, e.g. by offering equal time to all team members.
- Establishes role clarity for each professional in the context of what the team is trying to achieve so that every professional's unique contribution is spelt out.
- Ensures the knowledge base of each professional is respected and that its core points are incorporated into the team's operational knowledge base.
- Actively works to resolve any inter-professional conflict as soon as it appears.

Strong leaders of partnerships also demonstrate:

- Entrepreneurial leadership (innovation)
- Professional leadership (work done properly or correctly)
- Cultural leadership (creating a shared sense of purpose)
- Emotional and psychological leadership (engagement).

It is important to be realistic about leadership and management. Most of the time it is messy. It is impossible to be super-competent, due to the sheer number and type of demands faced. Things often go wrong: some could have been prevented, others couldn't. Events or situations can cause days, weeks or months of corrosive worry and pressure for those responsible, even if the events or situations were beyond their control as many are. Managing a merged organisation, or managing in one, can equally add to the complexity quotient facing all social care managers (see Chapter 7 for comment on the rise in tasks all managers are having to deal with). Structures and personnel may be unfamiliar, and from being a member of a majority culture, you can suddenly find yourself in an uncomfortable minority, unfamiliar with the language, the values and the processes. This is another reason for adequate preparation and lead in time for a major change associated with a new structure and roles.

The infrastructure of partnerships

Governance

Good governance is central to promoting justifiable public confidence in an organisation, especially at a time of increasing cynicism about public services, and concerns about propriety in a post-Enron world which understandably led to more rigorous reporting requirements, to and by boards and executive teams. The public have a general right and people who use services have a particular right to value for money, good decision-making and high quality services. Of the many good governance checklists available for organisations to use, those by the Audit Commission, the Charity Commission, the Foundation for Good Governance and the NUS are useful examples.

Whilst operational staff sometimes claim they cannot move for inspectors, auditors, scrutiny committees, accreditation and licensing systems and boards, people who use services need a range of built-in checks and balances to be operating well around the clock, including safe whistleblowing procedures. A great number of social care disasters-in-the-making have been avoided as a direct result of whistleblowers. Even though many have gone unreported and unrecorded because of the sensitivity of the whistleblower's position, more serious problems in the future have often been prevented. For some service users though, it is already far too late. In October 2005, I met a 25-year-old woman who disclosed she was sexually abused in a children's home in the mid 1990s. She did not want action taken. She had far more pressing problems. Often, by the time a scandal is retrospectively uncovered, it is too late for the victims. In 1980, *The Irish Independent* ran the first story about child abuse in the Kincora Children's Home, after two social workers had blown the whistle that a paedophile ring was operating in children's homes in Northern Ireland, with links to businessmen and paramilitary groups. It was subsequently discovered that children had been talking about their abuse since 1967, so it took 13 years for it to be acted upon (Moore 1996). In 2006, the Childrens Society, Torbay Council and Devon and Cornwall Constabulary, wrote a new missing persons protocol, containing the automatic offer to a young person of an independent interview when they returned or were found, as feedback from young people was that no-one was listening to why they were running away. Local agencies need to work together constantly to review the relevance of their current operations to today's circumstances (see 'Some who go missing, stay missing' box).

New legislation such as freedom of information (FOI) legislation places an emphasis on citizen's rights to know what is going on at all times, even if it remains hard to penetrate the inner citadels of organisations. More positively, partnerships have a chance as well as a responsibility to demonstrate they take governance seriously by working within the key principle of good governance being the 'involvement of society in the process of governing' (Pierre and Peters 2000). This means setting an example in everything from

Some who go missing, stay missing

'When Andrew Smith died, aged 40, nobody noticed' (Leve 2007). Smith had gradually become disconnected from his family, had no friends, and did not work. He was fostered at six months old, and grew up with foster parents until he left home. At 18 he traced and met his birth mother, but contact was not maintained. In the years before his death, he became unwell with type-1 diabetes. The coroner could not tell if he died of this, or simply lost the will to live, a syndrome not confined to the very old. Was being fostered the key factor? Did he grow up never quite feeling connected? Hampshire County Council had lost his file, but even if his childhood was catalogued, it is unlikely this question could have been answered. In 2004, seven million people in the UK lived alone, four times as many as in 1961. By 2021, 37 per cent of all households will be made up of people who live alone. It is hard enough responding to people who do reach out in different ways, it is near impossible to reach those who deliberately put themselves beyond all help.

robust schedules of delegation to demonstrate where decisions are taken, to being carbon neutral and putting in place, monitoring and evaluating a good sustainability strategy. Some Partnership Boards now insist members sign a Membership Agreement or Compact Agreement, to deepen their engagement and commitment (see below), although such increasingly popular signing-up is only a paper exercise if all the other constraints upon partnership working discussed in this book are present.

Partnerships make organisational transparency more complex as it is harder to see the audit and decision trails in a partnership, even if the statutory accountabilities of individual partners remain separate. 'Partnerships present a challenge to the principles of public sector corporate governance' (Sullivan and Skelcher 2002), and it is important to develop joint governance systems to compensate, such as joint audit committees, joint corporate risk management committees and shared risk registers. Care has to be taken not to create an unduly complex governance structure, with a multiplicity of boards which then prove hard to co-ordinate, as in solving one problem, a worse problem can be created.

Complaints handling and redress needs to be 'central in the governance of partnerships', as people who use services often lack information about how to register a complaint. This is exacerbated by confusion amongst staff and public about how the complaints-handling process works, including what protections staff have against malicious or gratuitous complaints and complainants (Redmond 2007).

Oxfordshire Safeguarding Children Board

Membership Agreement

1. Duty to Safeguard

This membership agreement represents an agreement between Oxfordshire County Council as the body with the statutory duty under Section 13(1) Children Act 2004 and its Board partners as defined in Section 13(3) of the Act, together with relevant persons and bodies as defined in Section 13(4) to (6) of the Act. It also recognises the explicit two way duty of co-operation between the Council as the Children's Services Authority establishing Oxfordshire Safeguarding Children Board (OSCB) and each Board partner, as set out in Section 13(7) of the Act.

2. Purpose

The agencies and organisations represented on the OSCB share a statutory commitment under the Children Act 2004 to co-operate and work together to safeguard and promote the welfare of children.

It is each member's responsibility and duty to contribute to steering the strategic direction of the OSCB and to ensure implementation of both Working Together Guidance and Standard 5 of the National Framework.

The OSCB is responsible for co-ordinating local agencies' arrangements and has a collective responsibility for ensuring the effectiveness of local arrangements and services of all agencies working with children in Oxfordshire:

To focus agency activity on delivering improved outcomes for children as defined in the priorities outlined in the Children and Young People's Plan.

To ensure strong and effective inter-agency arrangements proactively to co-ordinate the delivery of safeguarding arrangements through the implementation of the OSCB strategy and supporting plans.

3. Expectations of Members

All board members will share the responsibility for ensuring that the OSCB objectives are delivered. Members of each individual sub-group will be responsible and accountable for agreeing their terms of reference and supporting plans within their remit.

Each Board partner accepts the responsibility to:

OSCB Membership Agreement
1

- Ensure their agency is represented with 100% attendance of which no more than 20% should be by an alternative named representative.

- Be responsible for their agency's contribution to safeguarding children whether this be agency resources, financial, human or in kind, and to ensure they are utilised to meet OSCB objectives. Any shortfalls should be brought to the attention of their agency and the Board.

- Act as a channel of communication between their own agency and the Board and to be the named advocate for safeguarding in all matters relating to the OSCB within their agency/professional body.

- Accept responsibility for monitoring the effectiveness of arrangements, to contribute to and examine regular updates, data and analysis on individual and joint agency performance.

4. Terms and Conditions

It is expected that the OSCB representatives will be senior managers within their organisation. Members should be able to commit their agency/professional body to joint working and in some cases allocate and/or reshape resources to support the work of the OSCB.

It is expected that named representatives will normally serve a minimum of three years on the OSCB. Any extension of this will be discussed and negotiated with the OSCB Chair or Business Manager.

No fees will be paid by the OSCB for agency time or expenses for attendance at meetings. Where exceptions exist this will be defined in the subgroup/business plan and negotiated with the OSCB Business Manager.

Agencies will be expected to respect any OSCB shared information as confidential and will be expected to sign a confidentiality agreement.

All agencies will ensure that their nominated statutory or non statutory members have an up to date, clear Enhanced Criminal Records Bureau (CRB) Check.

Signed   Agency

Agency representative OSCB

OSCB Membership Agreement
2

Figure 5.3 Oxfordshire Safeguarding Children Board Membership Agreement

Good 'partnership working etiquette' is an essential component of good governance, particularly about how to behave. Appropriate behaviours can be written into a Code of Partnership Conduct, which can be retained as part of a publicly available governance document pack. This can be applied to all sets of working relationships within a partnership, including with trade unions, where 'behaviours such as joint commitment, joint recognition of each side's legitimate interests, loyalty to each other and joint commitment to operating in a transparent manner are important in maintaining partnership working' (Luckhurst 2004).

A rigid defensive approach to governance can lead to petty parochialism – *my* school, *my* team, *my* budget. Establishing detailed governance structures for lots of small organisations within an alliance can lead to fresh silos, and a reluctance to collaborate, especially if governors or non-executive directors have a vested interest in maintaining their own organisation and see no collaborative advantage in partnership working (Huxham and Vangen 2005). This process can be eased by involving people who use services or their representatives in governance structures, including on boards, as the 'end user' can be a long way away from the rarefied atmosphere and dialogue at senior board and executive levels.

Governance is exercised on behalf of people who need and use services, to ensure they are receiving the service they should be, and on behalf of taxpayers, to ensure public money is well spent. At a conference of Directors of Social Services and local politicians in charge of social services in England and Wales a few years ago, a young woman stood up and asked, 'how many children have you got?' Several directors and lead members put their hands up when she shouted out '1': more put them up when she shouted '2'; then fewer and fewer until she got to '7' when no-one put their hands up. She then berated them for not including all children looked after in their council. The correct answer, she suggested, is the total number of children in care in your council! One young person in care said to me, 'I know my social worker cares for me, because she sent me a postcard when she went on holiday'. Good parenting of children looked after means good parenting by the local authority as a corporate parent, good parenting by foster carers and good parenting in loco parentis by school teachers – *mass corporate parenting*.

Good governance should also be extended to staff rights. For example, under health and safety legislation, each employee on an organisation's Disabled Person's Register should have a personal evacuation plan in the event of the building she or he works in needing to be evacuated, and a personal access plan to buildings used for training events – small points, but big issues to the staff members concerned, who are often institutionally forgotten.

IT in partnership working

The core relationship between government and individual citizens in the future is likely to be one of information partners. The ServiceCanada website, in English and French, has all public services in Canada within easy 'e-reach', including online services and service access points in one place in a well organised website, far ahead of most other countries. The Seattle Community Network is a free public-access computer network for exchanging and accessing information, accessible from public places and attempting to link users into a wider set of databases. The UK's Direct.Gov.uk is seeking to achieve the same coverage, public access and awareness, and within the UK, most organisations are developing an online interactive capacity to communicate with their customers or end users. For example, HMRC are developing enhanced communication and interaction with both end users and intermediaries such as accountants about tax returns, and HM Land Registry is developing e-conveyancing to facilitate electronic access to details on the register by conveyancing professionals.

Technology increases the possibilities of reciprocal service arrangements. The voluntary organisation for families, Relate, has a national call centre with therapeutically trained call-centre counsellors, Relate Response, which can switch calls with the Child Maintenance and Enforcement Commission (CMEC), formerly the Child Support Agency, when CMEC feels the relationship problem at the heart of a financial dispute between a resident and non-resident parent needs specialist counselling.

IT is transforming service delivery. Kooth (see Chapter 2), through a public/private partnership, provides a transactional online service for young people offering professional counselling and advice, supported by an early intervention team offering rapid face-to-face contact if required (www.kooth. com).

Though not a service industry, partnerships with internet providers are yielding results. Bebo has 8 million users, 42 per cent of whom are between 13 and 30. MySpace has 177 million members, with 320,000 signing up every day. Unsurprisingly, a partnership between Bebo, the NSPCC and Childline led to far more take-up and engagement by children with campaigns.

Between 2001 and 2003, No Panic, a small voluntary group in Shropshire, working in partnership with another group, Truce, and Shropshire Community Network, ran 150 self-facilitating teleconferencing 'recovery' groups for isolated people with anxiety-related disorders, and has set up follow on befriending groups.

Satnav/GPRS systems are being used by many community support teams to help locate someone with dementia who's lost, allowing a degree of safe wandering. This certainly has advantages over the method adopted by John Bayley with his wife, the novelist Iris Murdoch, who had dementia. He pinned her nightie to him as they slept so he'd be alerted if she wandered off (Bayley 2002).

Advanced assistive technology is making community care safer, in ways such as a local care provider using broadband to communicate directly with people in their own home through their television sets, to check on their safety and needs, and travel training for people with learning disabilities using handheld computers. A partnership today can be via a speech-recognition computer program, which is enabling someone with profound multiple disabilities to communicate for the first time. A snakes and ladders game with a raised surface and a chunky wooden version of noughts and crosses can help deaf blind service users feel more comfortable as well as help assessors to assess need more accurately.

Good IT can also support effective operational work. It can keep front-line staff in isolated locations like lighthouse keepers, coastguards and British immigration officers in Sangatte, France in touch with colleagues – small numbers of staff but in crucial roles.

In many ways, the technology is moving faster than those using it. Technology continues to change rapidly, with blade-frame technology now able to replace 100 servers with a single server using 'virtualisation' technology. Hampshire County Council has developed a 'partnership portal' and West Lancashire District Council has introduced a revolutionary microwave CCTV used by US special forces. New collaborative technologies are coming onto the market weekly, like software that can instantly translate a document into another language for people needing services for whom English is not a first language, allowing agencies to dispense with expensive manual translation services.

As a rule of thumb, 20 per cent of IT problems are with the technology, and 80 per cent are with the users, including problems with data security and data losses. Disputes or dilemmas about information sharing are one of the biggest cultural constraints to partnership working (Richardson and Asthana 2006). Nearly all partnerships are struggling to build shared databases and common datasets, and many programmes are limited through a lack of ability to analyse the most basic acts of joint working, including common units of management information and other data inter-operability problems. A common system platform is needed, with system architecture evolving over a period of time, otherwise there are too many levels of complexity, and an unnecessarily large number of staff are needed to maintain and forge links between separate systems. Many new information sharing projects are in the development stage, such as a secure communication link between three government departments (Department for Children, Schools and Families (DCSF), Department of Communities and Local Government (DCLG) and the Ministry of Justice (MOJ)), and local authorities, which will speed up a number of transactions and processes between central and local government.

New national databases are also being developed, based on the questionable premise that information technology holds many of the answers to a lack of effective communication between professionals, even though case histories show that no system is 100 per cent foolproof technically and its accuracy will be a lot less than 100 per cent if the staff across agencies are not trained and not fully committed. One such database is Contactpoint, in which every child in England will have their own unique identifying number. As

Lyons speculated, 'Organisations of many kinds will know us only as coded sequences of numbers and letters' (Lyon 1994).

Boyle and Leadbetter are adamant that existing systems in themselves, including registration and inspection arrangements, do not adequately protect vulnerable people (Boyle and Leadbetter 1998). Individual organisations have to take an extra and more personal level of responsibility for ensuring that they apply adequate safeguards.

References

4Ps, 2008, *PFI Operational Project Review: Adult Social Care, 2008*, London: Public Private Partnerships Programme.

Allen, E., 2002, *Starting to Modernise: Managing Strategic Service Delivery Partnerships*, London: New Local Government Network.

Atkinson, M., Wilkin, A., Stott, A., Doherty, P. and Kinder, K., 2002, *Multi-agency Working: A Detailed Study*, Slough: National Foundation for Educational Research.

Audit Commission, 2007, *Out of Authority Placements for Special Educational Needs*, London: Audit Commission.

Bamford, J., Gomes Casseres, B. and Robinson, M., 2003, *Mastering Alliance Strategy*, San Francisco: Jossey-Bass.

Bate, P., Khan, R. and Pye, A., 2000, 'Towards a culturally sensitive approach to organisational structuring: where organisation design meets organisation development', *Organisation Science*, 11(2): 197–211.

Bayley, J., 2002, *Iris: A Memoir of Iris Murdoch*, London: Abacus.

Boyle, M. and Leadbetter, M., 1998, *Enough is Enough*, London: Association of Directors of Social Services.

Cabinet Office, 2004, *Trade Union and Employee Involvement in Public Sector Reform*, (prepared for the Public Service Forum), London: Cabinet Office.

Cavanagh, J., Business Development Director of the National Audit Office, 2007, quoted in *The Observer*, 19 August.

Chambers, E., 2004, *Roots for Radicals Organising for Power Action and Justice*, London: Continuum International Publishing.

Clarke, M., 1998, Co-government – governance and the European Union: A discussion of co-government, *Local Governance*, 24(1): 3–21.

Collins, J., 2006, *Good to Great and the Social Sectors*, New York: Random House.

Douglas, A., June 2002, 'Is anybody out there: a study of recruitment and retention in social care in London', supplementary report for the *Care in the Capital Campaign*.

Drexler, E., 1995, 'Introduction to Nanotechnology', in M. Krummenacker and J. Lewis (eds), *Prospects in Nanotechnology: Towards Molecular Manufacturing (Proceedings of the First General Conference on Nanotechnology: Development, Applications and Opportunities)*, New York: Wiley and Sons.

Essex County Council, 2006, *Establishing Local Integrated Teams in Children's Services*, Cabinet Report, 24 October, Chelmsford: Essex County Council.

Elbeik, S. and Thomas, M., 1998, *Project Skills*, London: Butterworth Heinemann.

Flanagan, R., 2008, *The Review of Policing: Final Report*, London: Home Office.

Fletcher, K., 2006, *Partnerships in Social Care: A Handbook for Developing Effective Services*, London: Jessica Kingsley.

Frost, N., 2005, *Professionalism, Partnership and Joined-Up Thinking*, Totnes: Research in Practice.

Glendinning, C., Halliwell, S., Jacobs, S., Rummery, K. and Tyrer, J., 2000, 'New kinds of care, new kinds of relationships: how purchasing services affects relationships in giving and receiving personal assistance', *Health and Social Care in the Community*, 8(3): 201–11.

George, M., 2002, *Lean Six Sigma*, New York: McGraw Hill.

Ghosn, C., 2007, quoted in *The World in 2006*, London: The Economist.

Glisson, C. and Hemmelgarn, A., 1998, 'The effects of organisational climate and interorganisational co-ordination on the quality and outcomes of children's services systems?', *Child Abuse and Neglect*, 22: 401–21.

Goffman, E., 1970, *Asylums: Essays on the Social Situation of Mental Patients and Other Inmates*, Harmondsworth: Pelican Press.

Grayling, A., 2001, *The Meaning of Things*, London: Weidenfeld and Nicholson.

Greig, R. and Poxton, R., 2001, 'From joint commissioning to partnership working – will the new policy framework make a difference?', *Managing Community Care*, 9(4): 32–8.

Ham, C., 2008, *Financial Times*, 8 January.

Hudson, B., 2006, 'Integrated team working: you can get it if you really want it', *Journal of Integrated Care*, 14(1):13–22.

Hudson, B., Exworthy, M., Peckham, S. and Callaghan, G., 1999, *Locality in Partnerships: The Early Primary Care Group Experience*, Leeds: Nuffield Institute for Health, University of Leeds.

Huxham, C. and Vangen, S., 2005, *Managing to Collaborate*, London: Routledge.

IPA (Involvement and Participation Association), 2001, *Sharing the Challenges Ahead: Informing and Consulting With Your Workforce*, London: IPA.

IPA (Involvement and Participation Association) and Unions 21, 2005, *Moving Partnership on*, London: IPA.

IVAR (Institute for Voluntary Action Research, 2008, *Key Findings on Voluntary Sector Mergers*, 2008, London: IVAR.

Jones, S., 2006, *Antonio Gramsci*, Critical Thinkers Series, Oxon: Routledge.

Kotter, J., 2006, *Our Iceberg is Melting*, Basingstoke: Macmillan.

KPMG, 2006, *The Morning After: Driving for Post-deal Success*, London: KPMG.

Langdon, D. and Rawlinson, S., 2006, 'Procurement – construction management', *Building Magazine*, 1 September.

Leutz, W., 1999, 'Five laws for integrating medical and social services: lessons from the US and UK', *Millbank Quarterly*, 77 (1): 77–110.

Leve, A., 2007, 'Broken pieces of a lost life', *Sunday Times Magazine*, 2 September.

Liker, J., 2004, *The Toyota Way: 14 Management Principles from the World's Greatest Manufacturer*, New York: McGraw-Hill.

Luckhurst, D., 2004, *Partnership Working: A Practitioner's Guide*, London: Involvement and Participation Association.

Lyon, D., 1994, *The Electronic Eye: The Rise of the Surveillance Society*, Minneapolis, MN: University of Minnesota Press.

Malik, S., 2007, 'The making of a terrorist', *Prospect Magazine*, June.

Marchant, R., 2008, *What Makes a Successful Public Private Partnership*, Portland, OR: Solace Foundation.

Martin, S., 2006, *Public Service Improvement: Policies, Progress and Prospects*, Oxon: Routledge.

McCann, J. and Gray, B., 1986, 'Power and collaboration in human service domains', *International Journal of Sociology and Social Policy*, 6: 58–67.

McCormack, M., 1994, *What They Don't Teach You at Harvard Business School*, New York: Profile Business.

Moore, C., 1996, *The Kincora Scandal: Political Cover-up and Intrigue in Northern Ireland*, Blackrock: Marino Books.

National Audit Office, 2007, *Improving Corporate Functions Using Shared Services*, London: NAO.

National Audit Office, 2008, *Making Operational Changes in PFI Projects*, London: NAO.

National College for School Leadership, 2007, *What We Know About School Leadership*, Nottingham: NCSL.

National College for School Leadership, 2006, *Seven Strong Claims About Successful School Leadership*, Nottingham: NCSL.

O'Cinneide, M. and Keane, M.J., 1990, 'Applying strategic planning to local economic development: the case of Connemara Gaeltacht, Ireland', *Town Planning Review*, 61(4): 475–86.

Peck, E. and Crawford, A., 2004, *Culture in Partnerships: What do We Mean by it and What Can We do about it?'*, London: Integrated Care Network.

Peck, E., Gulliver, P. and Towell, D., 2002, *Modernising Partnerships: An Evaluation of Somerset's Innovations in the Commissioning and Organisation of Mental Health Services*, London: Institute of Applied Health and Social Policy, Kings College.

Peschanki, D., Durand, Y., Veillon, D., Ory, P., Azema, J.P., Frank, R., Eichart, J. and Marechal, D., 1988, *Collaboration and Resistance: Images of Life in Vichy France 1940–1944*, New York: Harry N. Abrams.

Pierre, J. and Peters, G., 2000, *Governance Politics and the State*, Basingstoke: Macmillan.

Redmond, T., 2007, *Local Partnerships and Citizen Redress*, London: Local Government Ombudsman.

Reeves, B., Malone, T. and O'Driscoll, T., 2008, 'Leadership's online labs', *Harvard Business Review*, May.

Richardson, S. and Asthana, S., 2006, 'Interagency information sharing in health and social care services: the role of professional culture', *British Journal of Social Work*, 36: 657–69.

Riedel, G., 2006, quoted in 'Understanding collaboration', *Financial Times*, 10 November, p. 5.

Social Exclusion Task Force, 2008, *Think Family*, London: Social Exclusion Task Force in the Cabinet Office.

Springett, J., 1995, *Intersectoral Collaboration: Theory and Practice*, Occasional paper, Liverpool: Institute of Health, John Moores University.

Sudarsanam, S., 2003, *Creating Value from Mergers and Acquisitions: The Challenges*, New York: Prentice Hall.

Sull, D., 2001, 'Success flows from business development', *Mastering Management, Financial Times*, 15 January.

Sullivan, H. and Skelcher, C., 2002, *Working Across Boundaries: Collaboration in Public Services*, Basingstoke: Palgrave, Basingstoke.

Swann, P., Director of the Tavistock Institute, 2007, interview in *The Guardian*, 17 January.

Taylor, A., Harrison, R., Mann, G. and Murphy, M., 2003, *Partnership Made Painless: A Joined-up Guide to Working Together*, Lyme Regis: Russell House Publishing.

Taylor, M., 2008, *Brent Teaching PCT: Independent Management Review: Financial Management and Corporate Governance*, London: NHS.

Trinder, L. and Kellett, J., 2007, *The Longer Term Outcomes of In-Court Conciliation*, Ministry of Justice Research Series 15/07, London: Ministry of Justice.

Unison, 2007, *Integration of Health and Social Care Services: Organising Issues for Unison*, London: Unison.

Von Neumann, J. and Morgenstern, D., 1944, *Theory of Games and Economic Behaviour*, Princeton, NJ: Princeton University Press.

Voorhees, J., 2002, *Dialogue Sustained: The Multi-Level Peace Process and the Dartmouth Conference*, Washington, DC: United States Institute of Peace.

Walker, L.O. and Avant, K.C., 1995, *Strategies of Theory Construction in Nursing* (3rd edn), Norwalk, CT: Appleton and Lange.

Wenger, E., 1998, *Communities of Practice: Learning, Meaning and Identity*, Cambridge: Cambridge University Press.

Wenger, E., McDermott, R. and Snyder, W., 2002, *Cultivating Communities of Practice: A Guide to Managing Knowledge*, Boston, MA: Harvard Business School Press.

Wilson, A., 2005, *Virtual Politics: Faking Democracy in the Post-Soviet world*, New Haven, CT: Yale University Press.

6 Partnership working in practice

Key messages

- Each social care case should become a unique partnership with many people communicating and working together
- Assessments and care plans need to be evidence based, with the evidence gathered through skilled partnership working
- Social care needs the support of other agencies if it is to be able to do its job properly – no social care service is an island
- Multi-agency teams are now the norm: pretty soon there will be blanket coverage, an astonishing policy and practice shift within a generation
- The more complex the case, the more non-negotiable is partnership working

---

The purpose of partnership working in cases

Recent trends

The purpose of partnership working in cases is to ensure that a person's needs can be properly assessed, and that the right services are provided – and it cannot be done in the absence of partnerships. An assessment and care plan for someone with acute mental health problems will involve a social care worker spending time with the person needing a service, discussing the person with family and/or friends, in order to understand their perspective on what has been happening, and discussing the person's needs and any risks with professionals like a GP. To be successful, those conversations have to take place within a partnership framework if all involved are to be put at ease and to feel they are making a contribution to the potential service user's health and well-being.

Two recent trends are clear. The first is that there is more support 'out there' for children and adults in need from social care agencies and networks than ever before. For example, 87 per cent of Sure Start Children's Centres are working with childminders in their area, support that childminders will not have had before on that scale (http://www.ncma.org.uk/MainWebSite/Resources/Document/childrens_centres_research_08.doc). Increased funding to youth justice and substance misuse services has expanded the number of contracts to support many children and adults on the edge of care, psychiatric units or prison. However, whilst more vulnerable people are being supported and receiving a better service once they get into the system, those outside the system are receiving little if any help. They are also vulnerable adults with a significant level of unmet need (CSCI 2008), and the same can be said for children.

This is the gap which strong partnership working and joined-up services is attempting to close, particularly through expanding prevention and support services. Radical changes in working practices are the only way this gap can be bridged, and this is now realised by government (in England) in new statutory guidance on inter-agency co-operation in new children's trusts, which says 'the only way preventative and early intervention work will be successful is if the Children's Trust becomes the mainstream service' (Department for Children, Schools and Families 2008). This will entail a range of mainstream universal services taking on the vulnerability agenda, such as community schools (Bryan *et al.* 2006).

On the run, but with hope

Three children from Zanzibar, on the run since 1997, moved from Zanzibar, to Burundi and then to London. The mother was raped by soldiers and driven out of her village. Her husband was killed. They finally settled in London, playing cat and mouse with the police and immigration service for years. At the same time, the children, now 17, 12 and 5, were receiving a good education. Then they were discovered and deported. After the family were removed back to Dar es Salaam, homeless and without resources, all their family in East Africa now dead, the 17-year-old was about to be married off to a 40-year-old man who had promised to pay the upkeep of her mother and siblings. She rebelled and, still in touch with friends at school in a British city, and supported by the local Swahili Association, arrangements were made for her to fly back to the UK to continue her education. This was endorsed by the local education authority, despite the young woman's immigration status being unclear. The case also shows that support for individuals from minority ethnic communities is usually stronger than for those communities as a whole. Once an individual person becomes real for people, equality is easier.

Clara: get me to the court on time

Clara was seventeen and three-quarter years old when she suddenly announced that she wanted to be adopted by the foster parents she had lived with for three years. She said she needed security in her life, and did not want to be an adult without any legal ties to her parents – her birth parents were both dead. Normally, the adoption process from assessment to legal order would take at least a year to complete, with its various stages inside the adoption agency and in court. However, at a case conference, all professionals involved decided to hold a special one off Adoption Panel and Court Hearing specifically to consider the adoption assessment, the matching of Clara with her adopters, the past family issues including representations from her birth relatives, and most importantly, the needs wishes and feelings of Clara herself. She was adopted with three days to spare.

   This happy ending shows what can be done by making the process fit the service user, not the other way round.

The second trend is that most agencies are making great efforts to implement the partnership working requirement, despite what at times seem insurmountable difficulties.

The two examples in the boxes show how statutory and voluntary organisations can work together to enhance the future prospects of two 17-year-old young women. These are genuinely user-centred services, where the partnership with the person using the service is at the heart of the case and casework process (see Chapter 3).

Partnerships in assessment

'If your photographs aren't good enough, you're not close enough'.
(Robert Capa 1942)

Over the course of a year, one 83-year-old woman in London suffered 57 falls and had to deal with 14 different health and social care professionals. It was 12 months before someone asked why, rather than how, she fell. A lop-sided mattress was rolling her out of bed. Once the cause was established, something could be done about it. It just took someone to ask the right question. She was unable to speak up for herself.

   Assessment should be proportionate to the problems being addressed. Some needs are simple, and can be self-assessed. At the other end of the spectrum, a full joint assessment of need is needed by a team of professionals working together.

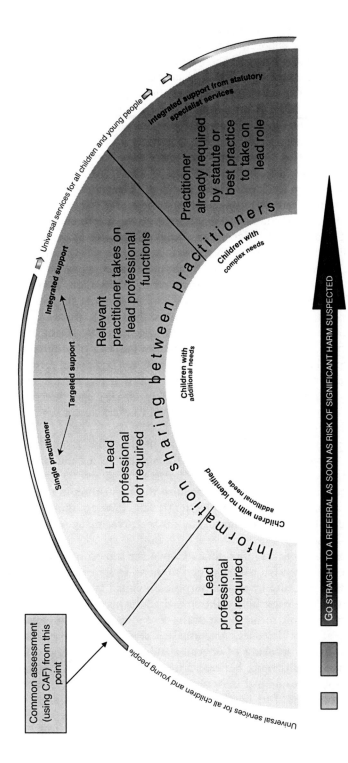

Figure 6.1 The common assessment framework

The Government's framework for this is the common assessment framework (CAF) for children and the single assessment process (SAP) for adults, derived from the National Service Framework (NSF) for older people, and used in conjunction with FACS (Fair Access to Care Services). The CAF brought together other bespoke assessment systems like Asset (Youth Offending Teams), APIR (Connexions), and the educational statementing process, to be a multi-agency front-door assessment underpinned by good partnership working.

Despite the fact that these new frameworks were universally welcomed, researchers were soon concluding that 'use of this (CAF) framework had made no difference to the level of joint working' (Cleaver *et al.* 2004).

'Assessment' has come to mean either an *assessment of risk* or an *assessment of need*. Both require a combination of information and intelligence gathering, and a set of professional judgements about the relative importance and priority of different pieces of information. Journalists call this the 'jigsaw effect', which is where disparate details about an issue appear in different media over time, allowing the piecing together of information. This is often only possible after an event or incident, where subsequent inquiries often point to basic faults in the assessment and analysis of a situation. In the Cumbrian rail crash in 2007, one of three stretcher bars was missing and two others were fractured. Neither a visual assessment nor laser photography had picked this up. This shows how the simplest faults can be missed. A report by Network Rail concluded that two different inspection teams each assumed the other had carried out the necessary safety checks, and that personal disputes and communication problems between workers were a key factor in the misunderstanding (*Observer*, 26 August 2007).

Assessing risk in families, where harm is often not visible, is much harder. A boy with burns on his buttocks was the subject of a child protection investigation, until it was discovered the burns were caused by battery acid being absorbed into his skin as a caustic burn through sitting in the back of a car where a battery had been inadvertently left. Physical abuse was only discounted after laboratory testing of the car seat. Not many investigations would go to those lengths.

Accurate assessments are more difficult when the subject of an assessment is reluctant to describe what has happened to them. Despite improvements in assessment standards, and improved purpose-equipped facilities in which to conduct assessments, vulnerable children and adults may still be reluctant to tell their story, primarily through fear of the consequences or fear of personal disintegration if their defences, functional to coping with their situation, are breached. Kohli, speaking of unaccompanied asylum seeking children, describes this as the difference between a thin and a thick story. A thin story is a cover story, with minimal information given out or where a rehearsed or coached story is told to investigators or assessors. A thick story is the real story, which the child can only express when feeling secure and able to trust the adult or adults now looking after her or him (Kohli 2005). Kohli describes the care task as helping such children and young people with a 're-emergence of order, emotional recovery and establishment of the rhythm of ordinary life' (Kohli 2006).

The assessment process is fraught with the risk of multiple misunderstandings. When a question is asked, and the respondent does not realise they are about to incriminate themselves if they say the wrong thing, could social workers be accused of entrapment? Some prospective adopters claim this is the case because they were invited to speak about their personal relationships, their habits, lifestyle and views, without being made aware of how they would be consequentially judged. Of course the role of assessment in adoption is not to pry but to bring relevant issues out into the open and discuss them thoroughly. The impact of the assessor on the assessment also risks skewing a judgment, and sometimes 'the observer's simple act of looking at something will in some way immeasurably change it' (Polke 2003).

Whilst many people ask for help, and need to be assessed quickly and competently, other assessments can be compromised by lies and disinformation. Lie detectors are now used routinely in some assessment processes, for housing benefit claims for example, which use voice risk analysis technology. Assessors have to be on the look out for puffed up applications for benefits such as a blue badge through an overstatement of a level of disability. The key to an accurate assessment is to construct and then validate an evidence base. In some ways, social care investigations have become like police investigations, needing to rely on evidence which can be tested ultimately in a court of law, although in practice lower threshold tests have to be used if children and adults are to be properly safeguarded, as the evidence is frequently ambiguous.

As a practitioner, told many things by many service users, how do you distinguish between fact, urgent fact, exaggeration, fiction or delusion? Communication with captive service users who may need safeguarding can become ambivalent, with intrinsic trust difficulties that cannot be overcome. Assessing vulnerability can draw from unrelated disciplines such as espionage! The disinformation fed by an Iraqi engineer, codenamed Curveball, about Iraqi weapons of mass destruction prior to the Iraq War in 2003, had catastrophic consequences derived from a failure of assessment. 'Clandestine operatives are trained to spread falsehoods as part of their tradecraft. Intelligence agencies spin or hide the truth as a matter of policy and law. And spy services, even close allies, routinely conceal information from each other. In this case, the layers of secrecy and deception created a Rashomon effect: each group saw Curveball through a different lens. At the heart of the problem was a poor relationship between the German and American security agencies. 'There was visceral, mutual antagonism', a senior CIA official said, 'The BND doesn't like the CIA and vice versa' agreed a senior German intelligence officer. 'There is an adversarial relationship. Neither side trusts the other' (Drogin 2007).

Despite years of improving guidelines and training programmes for social care staff, many social care cases, when retrospectively de-briefed, continue to attract major criticisms. To quote from one serious case review (2007):

- 'serious communication issues both between agencies and between the two boroughs where the family lived'
- 'a lack of co-ordination between Children's Services and Adult Services'
- 'the assessments were too adult-focused and not sufficiently child-focused'
- 'the professional network was polarised'.

Boys who offend: understanding why can save their lives

Martin, a 14-year-old boy I worked with in 1982, was the scourge of the local police, and he became a priority case of mine. He was a persistent young offender before the term was invented. On one appearance before a Juvenile Court for taking and driving away a car (TDA), he asked for 123 similar offences to be taken into consideration. It turned out he was personally responsible for 60 per cent of TDAs in the local area over the previous few months. One year and hundreds of offences later, he told me had been seriously sexually abused within his family over a period of years when he was younger. It had stopped when he grew big enough to defend himself, although living at home made him permanently angry and upset.

Twenty-five years later, in 2007, a Serious Case Review (SCR) by Lancashire's Safeguarding Children Board, condemned the youth justice system for treating another 14-year-old, Adam Rickwood, as a tearaway who should be locked up rather than a vulnerable child needing care. Painful restraint techniques, such as the double basket hold, thumb distraction, rib distraction and nose distraction, were at the centre of criticisms. Adam killed himself in a Young Offender Institution (YOI), a day after receiving a sharp upward strike to the nose in the nose distraction restraint method, for refusing to go to his room. Adam had a history of self-harm but his risk assessment file was wrongly closed 11 days before his death. The report criticised a lack of information-sharing between agencies prior to his entry to custody.

The case helped to force a change in the machinery of government to bring the management of youth justice more into the remit of the Secretary of State for Children, Schools and Families, so that children who can offend can be treated as children first, and offenders second, through a dual key arrangement between the two respective secretaries of state.

Many other vulnerable groups have unrecognised mental health problems and in dire need of a partnership working model to support them, such as women in prison.

These risks of making a serious mistake should not detract from the need to work in partnership with people who need or use services even in the most hostile of circumstances. That is when teamwork is especially important, to give workers peer support and a second opinion under pressure. As Calder says, 'assessment is a process designed to inform the development of plans to improve the situation that gave rise to concern in the first instance' (Calder 2004). Calder distinguishes between questioning, exchange and procedural models, in which only the exchange model is a partnership model of assessment (Calder and Hackett 2003).

Joint assessments, like the Single Assessment Process, benefit from parallel development work and joint training. For instance, in using a shared assessment tool for older people in Scotland, nursing staff tended to over-state the need for further intervention and social care staff to under-state it (Eccles 2008). Calibration exercises at an early stage of implementation helped to produce convergence between the respective professional thresholds.

Partnerships in care management

The UK is unique in that it prioritises assessment over help or treatment. Many people receive an assessment of their needs but then never receive a service that might help them. For example, 46 per cent of parents subject to a child protection investigation said they didn't understand why they were being investigated and 69 per cent of parents said that lack of support exacerbated their difficulties (source: Family Rights Group). An unintended consequence of the extra bureaucratic burden of lengthy assessment processes is the risk of creating a new generation of 'desktop social workers', ticking boxes on an endless supply of unnecessarily long and repetitive forms.

Good practice example of integrated working

NCH Sure Start Exeter has pioneered an innovative parent-infant mental health service, that includes a parent–infant mental health specialist using CARE index training for staff. The group meets the needs of parents arising from CARE Index assessment and a post natal depression group. The project is currently piloting a parent–infant mental health model for Exeter Primary Care Trust, which will roll out across Exeter and through the Children's Trust to the rest of Devon. This whole programme response to preventative parent-infant mental health promotion in partnership with statutory agencies (health visitors, midwives, adult services and Sure Start Children's Centres staff) includes universal attachment surveillance through health visiting.

A written inter-agency case agreement to support and protect Child G (aged 2)

Core group

Social worker, family support team
Social worker, community mental health team (CMHT)
Health Visitor
SureStart worker
Family centre worker
Childminder
Mother
Maternal grandmother
Maternal grandmother's support worker

Examples of responsibilities of core group members

Social worker's responsibilities

1   To offer support and advice to mother and child
2   To co-ordinate and liaise with members of the core group about child G's safety and well-being
3   To visit mother and child at least every month
4   To liaise with probation about the child's father's release from prison

CMHT social worker's responsibilities

1   To visit mother fortnightly
2   To monitor changes in medication, particularly the recent reduction in anti-psychotic medication
3   To liaise with the consultant psychiatrist regarding any issues with medication
4   To support mother with confidence building and self esteem
5   To liaise with the social worker about any issues of concern

Health visitor's responsibilities

1   To continue to monitor Child G's health, development and progress
2   To visit Child G or to see him at the clinic at least monthly
3   To liaise with the social worker about any issues of concern

SureStart worker's responsibilities

1 To continue to offer support via:
   a)mother and toddler group
   b)individual outreach support
   c) other courses: first aid, art, basic hygiene (see weekly timetable)
2 To liaise with the social worker about any issues of concern

Mother's responsibilities

1 To continue to co-operate with the agencies involved in the care of her son G
2 To inform the CMHT worker if she is feeling unwell, tired or starting to suffer psychotic symptoms
3 To remain living with her mother for the foreseeable future
4 To seek legal advice from a named solicitor about a non-molestation order in respect of the child's father

Maternal grandmother's responsibilities

1 To provide ongoing supervision of her daughter in her parenting of G
2 To contact the CMHT worker if her daughter has a relapse
3 To liaise with the social worker if she has any concerns about her daughter's care of her son G
4 To liaise with the social worker if she or her daughter experience any harassment or have any concerns about the child's father following his release from prison

Signed ....
Signed....................
Signed....................
Signed....................
Signed....................
Signed....................

This is not how it was meant to be. 'Services to individuals (should) flow from an initial multi-agency assessment of individual and family needs, and should be integrated in a way that makes sense to the family, for example through key working' (Audit Commission 2003). The example from an NCH project (see 'Good practice example of integrated working' box) shows how it is possible to combine an assessment framework with a treatment programme.

Care management, including case management, is the organisation and delivery of care to someone assessed as needing a service, subject to eligibility criteria being met, and care being available – two large buts. The divide between assessment and care management can never be a rigid one. Circumstances in cases change, sometimes without warning, so care management must include perpetual re-assessment.

An example of an integrated care pathway

An increasing number of care management approaches have been developed over the last decade. One such programme, Sapphic, the Southern Area Professional Partnership for Hearing Impaired Children, aims to provide an integrated service from diagnosis to the end of Key Stage 1: to co-ordinate services alongside the implementation of universal screening; to identify professional roles with individual children; and to develop and support pre-school groups. Their core group for planning meetings is a paediatrician, speech and language therapist, an advisory teacher, a unit teacher, a social worker for deaf children, an audiological nurse, and an educational psychologist. This is an example of an *integrated care pathway*.

Coping with frustration

Members of core groups can become frustrated if the lead agency, usually children's or adult services in the local authority, does not make resources available to implement a care plan, leading to a strained partnership between management and front-line staff, where front-line staff feel their responsibility towards an individual service user is being compromised (Harlow and Shardlow 2006). This can be helped by complete clarity about the expectations on each core group member, including family members (see 'A written inter-agency agreement' box on p. 164).

Caseloads that can never be closed

At the heart of all statutory caseloads are a group of cases that can never be closed – individuals whose needs for care or protection are so great that without constant or regular support and protection, the consequences for individuals in that particular family or social system could be grave. Many such cases are open to a group of local agencies for one or more decades. They are social care's 'frequent flyers' to use an NHS term for regular visitors

Partnerships across sectors

Using funding from the Department for Communities and Local Government to reduce youth homelessness, the counselling organisation Relate provides a therapeutic mediation service between landlords and tenants who are vulnerable adults. The premise of the programme is that a relationship issue often lies behind both the homelessness and any difficulties between the landlord and the tenant.

The Borders Agency is developing a Code of Practice for Keeping Children Safe, and has pledged itself to work with children within the Every Child Matters framework by aligning care and immigration assessments, and to train its staff accordingly. It is also introducing a new post of Chief Inspector of the Borders Agency to look at the agency's performance in relation to children.

My own organisation, Cafcass, developed a protocol with the Borders Agency to create a facility for joint discussion of cases, a protocol partly enabled by my previous working relationships with both the Chief Executive and the Children's Champion of the Agency. This example shows how the principles of social care legislation are being increasingly taken on by other organisations in related fields as part of their interpretation of a legislative duty or Government policy to work in partnership (Borders Agency 2008).

---

to accident and emergency departments. The management of this group of cases takes up a disproportionate amount of time and resources, but this is unavoidable as those service users with the highest statutory needs have to receive the highest priority. In England, three times more is spent on 60,000 looked-after children than on 400,000 children in need, but the priority still has to be those for whom the state is the 'corporate parent'.

Resource problems

Resources for priority groups are still too often holding resources, not therapeutic resources. Adolescents in care are still far too often living in holding placements at great expense which produce no clear benefit, and which are not set up to do so. The Mental Health Act Commission described overcrowded and dirty psychiatric units, 'rife with aggression and fear', despite the UK spending twice as much as most other EU countries on mental health, and despite funding to the NHS having trebled between 2002 and 2007 (Mental Health Act Commission 2006 and 2008). *Commissioning a Brighter Future* promises more emphasis and spend on much-wanted psychological therapies (Department of Health 2007).

Tanya's story

Tanya's parents divorced. She stayed with her mother in the north of England and her father returned to live in his extended family in the east Midlands. Tanya's mum had alleged she was sexually and physically abused by her father, but there was no evidence and both parents continued to fight over who should look after her and how much contact the non-resident parent should have. An adult psychiatrist reported that the mother was suffering from a long-standing paranoid disorder.

Tanya's Cafcass guardian instructed a consultant child psychiatrist who advised that Tanya should be placed in a neutral environment to facilitate a clearer assessment of her needs. The court made an interim care order to the north of England local authority and ordered reports from both local authorities where the parents lived. Tanya was placed in a short-term foster placement.

The northern local authority concluded that Tanya needed to be placed away from her mother, but were concerned that her relationship with her father was fragile. The east Midlands authority thought Tanya should live with her paternal family in their area, subject to a further assessment of her views and wishes. The child psychiatrist supported a change of residence for Tanya. Working with the two local authorities, the guardian facilitated child and family psychiatric help in the east Midlands and housing for Tanya and her father. The court made a residence order to the father, and Tanya went to live with him, supported by a family assistance order. She settled in well with her father and had a relaxed and positive relationship with him.

After the family assistance order expired, the local authority agreed to continue to offer Tanya and her father support under Section 17 of the Children Act 1989. A sad coda to this story is that Tanya's father died soon afterwards. She returned to live with her paternal grandparents and they have since obtained a special guardianship order, with the same guardian involved.

This case study is a good example of inter-agency co-operation between two local authorities, who were able to negotiate Tanya's transfer from interim care in one authority, to a family placement in another; the support of medical experts in giving independent expert advice; the local hospital in responding promptly to Tanya's needs following her arrival in the East Midlands; and the children's guardian in playing a co-ordinating role.

Multi-agency partnerships to support vulnerable children and young people

> 'There's no clearer revelation of a society's soul than the way it treats its children'.
>
> (Nelson Mandela).

The lengths to which professional staff will go to safeguard a child defy belief, just as a lack of due care when a child dies through professional negligence defies belief. Helen Thompson, a children's guardian, spoke to 56 nurses in a hospital to gain a rounded picture of the mother/child relationship for a young child with unexplained fractures. That effort needs highlighting. Partnership working on cases takes place day in, day out, without a fuss, often securing life-changing improvements for people (see 'Tanya's story' box).

Prevention strategies

We know that multi-professional working is a major solution to the problems facing children in care, children on the edge of care and children in need. The leaders of new children's trusts are beginning, at the time of writing, to consider how best to support these children and young people before major problems develop. For instance, Hammersmith and Fulham Council in west London are focusing on the services that would have been needed by young people who committed knife crimes including murder in the borough. They discovered that all the young people had been brought up by single mothers and assessed that the absence of fathers was a key issue in their lives. They put a prevention programme, SOS, in place, which is now being evaluated.

In Lincolnshire, Hill Holt Wood, a community woodland project, helps Lincolnshire Education Authority provide full-time education for youngsters permanently excluded from school, through a combination of educational and vocational training, which is cheaper than out of county alternatives. The scheme is helping with reducing crime and anti-social behaviour.

The political focus on integrated services is without doubt encouraging professional staff to work together on the ground more systematically. A Cafcass practitioner told me the story in the 'A start of a life?' box.

The 'team around this child' was impressive. However, so much remains to be done. For 56 per cent of looked-after children, no one attends speech days and under half of a child's carers attend parents' evenings (Barnardos 2006).

Many schools are becoming multi-agency schools (see Chapter 5, section on leadership). When I was a school governor in an inner London primary school, we found that the best way to help Turkish children with their learning was to put on programmes to help their fathers become more literate and numerate. As a direct result, these fathers engaged more with their children, especially with their homework tasks. The contribution parents can make

A start of a life?

Some children were moving a long way to live with adoptive parents. There was no life story material – mum had died, her house had been cleared out, dad was missing. I went to the school the children had been to two years previously to ask if there were any photos or memories. Not only did the teacher remember the oldest child, she was deeply committed to trying to help. She asked other children to bring in photos and organised a reunion and farewell do with old classmates. This meant that the oldest child was able to go back to the area of origin which he remembered where he had a positive experience of being remembered and valued. Hats off to the school staff – shows what can be done!

to supporting their child's education, by involvement and encouragement, invites us to think not just about high-quartile schools in performance terms, but also high-quartile parents. Children need both.

Many schools have a strong partnership with their pupils. In Middlesborough, 9-year-old class counsellors and peer bullying counsellors, having been bullied themselves, give lessons on how to avoid being bullied, and how, if you are a bully, to realise the impact of what you do. Many schools, supported by the Anti-Bullying Alliance, have programmes in place which have dramatically reduced the incidence of bullying. In 2007, St Benedict's Comprehensive, Colchester, in Essex, had bully-free forms for the previous five years following a major internal partnership programme. 'I'm no longer a bully. I understand how she feels' – the words of a child who had been through the Toronto Roots of Empathy programme, applied in a Scottish school. One in three young people experience date violence and young women in Surrey, supported by Surrey County Council and Young Voice, produced a handbook and DVD, *Where is the Love?* to draw attention to the issue (Young Voice 2006).

Personal development has also been enhanced for Portugese children in south London through a multi-agency partnership, whose value statement is: 'From small acorns, trees grow', or in Portugese, 'De pequenino se torce o pepino'. The purpose of the partnership, between Sure Start Stockwell, London South Bank University, Lambeth Education Service, Sir Walter St Johns Charity, The Peter Minet Trust and the Walcot Educational Foundation, was to help Portugese/English children become fluently bi-lingual. 'Speaking Portugese at home is the best start you can give your child. The best way of helping with language development is talking to them all the time' (local partnership theme).

Joint working within children's services is likely to become more successful over the next few years, as all local agencies become more aware of, and enthused about, the children's trust model. Barnet Council's Education Champions scheme, introduced in 2004, in which senior managers mentor individual children looked after in their own authority, had by 2007 led to the proportion of children who sat at least one GCSE increasing from 64 per cent to 69 per cent and the percentage who achieved five or more A–C grades going up from 10 per cent to 23 per cent. This was double the national average for looked after children, whose starting point is often lower than average due to previous adverse family circumstances.

The raising of the participation age in education to 17 from 2013 and 18 from 2015

The last time this happened was in 1972, and a change of this magnitude can only happen once in a generation. Now there will be far more choice for young people – entry to learning programmes, the Foundation Learning Tier, Diplomas, GCSEs, A levels and apprenticeships. The language has changed (see Chapter 2). In 1972, the headline was the raising of the school-leaving age (ROSLA). Now it is softer, and expressed in terms of raising the participation age, and making an 'offer' to young people. The problems the new provision seeks to address are serious – to ensure young people in the UK can compete skills-wise in a global world, and to engage young people more, when there are clear signs of a lack of engagement of crucial groups especially in the Key Stage 3 years. The programme is a major partnership programme, as a powerful coalition of partners, including businesses offering accredited workplace training, will be needed to ensure enough 'offers' are made for the vision to be translated into reality within ten years.

Other changes between 1972 and 2008 are striking. In 1972, ministers did not 'meddle' in 'professional areas' like the curriculum. The curriculum is now hot political property, consistent with the politicisation of the professions, or the professionalisation and managerialisation of politics. In truth, the ownership of a social issue by politicians inevitably brings with it a desire for greater control, especially to make sure that good ideas are implemented rather than lost. Along with increased political ownership and investment, come tangible benefits for vulnerable groups (see below).

Many groups who never received skills training are now beginning to, such as young people in custody, even though as yet that training is not 'portable' in terms of transferable credits when they rejoin the outside world. The downside of political ownership is that an issue which is already hard for professionals to get to grips with, can be subjected to disorienting short-term political calculation.

From the top

In 2005, Ed Balls, a newly elected MP, became a champion of disabled children and their families when he met a group of parents at a special school in his constituency. Parents told him how difficult it was to access the services that their children needed and spoke frankly about how exhausting it was to provide care to a disabled child without a break. Spurred to action by the often negative experiences of parents and children across the country, he worked closely with the disabled children's lobby and other MPs in parliament, to raise the political profile of disabled children in government.

Eventually, after a joint HMT/DfES year-long review, Balls persuaded colleagues in the Treasury to agree new funding as part of the current Comprehensive Spending Review to transform services for disabled children across England over the next three years. This included £280 million to improve and expand provision of short breaks.

As Secretary of State for Children, Schools and Families, Balls continued to press for improved services to disabled children announcing a review of provision for children with speech and language difficulties and committing additional funding in the Children's Plan for children with special educational needs (SEN) and disabilities. Parents, campaigners and the charitable sector warmly welcomed Ball's commitment. In response, he made it clear that parents and disabled children and young people had a powerful impact on his thinking and that it was their collective voice, supported by advocates, that made the difference in securing new resources.

The stronger evidence base about what works in children's services, especially in family support, means resources can be targeted to schemes with proven track records like Family Nurse Partnership (FNP) programmes, a nurse-led intensive home visiting programme, now being piloted in ten sites across England as part of the Care Matters implementation plan (Katz and Pinkerton 2003).

Multiple agencies to tackle multiple problems

Two per cent of families, 140,000 across Britain, experience complex and multiple problems (Social Exclusion Unit 2008). At any one time, one per cent of young people aged between 16 and 18 are not in any form of education, employment or training. These families and young people continue to pose the greatest challenge of all to new children's trusts. They are a test of whether joint working can be effective with the most hard to reach groups. Not all current developments can automatically be relevant and helpful to these groups, many of whom are service users of heavy-end children's services in local authorities. For example, new extended schools with wrap around services may lack sufficient privacy for users of social care services. An example of a future programme being established to support this group of young people with the guarantee of a place in further education, employment or training, is profiled below, as an example of an issue that will be in the forefront of the next decade of joint working in children's services.

Multi-agency partnerships to support vulnerable adults

Partnership working is not new, and joint working, defined by two or more professionals from different disciplines discussing the care or treatment needs of a frail, ill or vulnerable person, has been the basis of social care since its origins. Social care is an eclectic profession and vocation, and has never laid claim to a knowledge base exclusively of its own. What it knows, it knows as part of a bigger picture, which it strengthens. An example of this is person-centred planning for people with learning disabilities. This movement began with advocates and people with learning disabilities themselves, supported by social workers. Over time, the medical model of caring for and treating people with learning disabilities was humanised. I remember in the 1980s a young woman with learning disabilities I worked with had toothache. Her dentist asked all the dental nurses in the surgery to come and hold her down while she had a filling. The young woman was scared of the dentist, but this did not warrant the use of restraint which would never have been carried out on a patient without learning disabilities.

The big shift in partnership working with vulnerable adults, particularly across health and social care, has been the replacement of the medical model in which people are just seen through their symptoms, to a social model or a socio-medical model, in which the cause as well as the symptoms are focused on, and, more than that, the person themselves is at the forefront of professional thinking.

The social model of disability enables onlookers to see the person, not the disability. In a service run by the charity I chair, the British Association of Adoption and Fostering (BAAF), called Be My Parent Online, videos of children with profound disabilities, including encrypted online clips, can be accessed by prospective adopters. The videos bring the child to life, compared to paper descriptions, which tend to emphasise their disabilities, not how the child adapts to them, and the help she or he needs. Bringing the child to life through a video profile helps the 'falling in love' process for the prospective carer. As Ivan Lewis, the Parliamentary Under Secretary of State for the Department of Health, said when speaking to the National Learning Disabilities Today Conference in November 2006, 'people with learning disabilities want a life, not a service'.

The 'multi-agency team around the vulnerable person or patient' concept is also being applied to adult services. Croydon Primary Care Trust has recreated a hospital ward environment in the community, a 'ward without walls', so that a multi-agency team now visits a patient in her or his own home, in the same way they would stand by a patient in a hospital bed to review care and treatment. A predictive risk modelling algorithm identifies which patients should be offered hospital admission. A virtual ward for children and a virtual hospice are being planned. Professionals use shared electronic notes, including a download of the GP record. A community matron co-ordinates care and calls in other professionals as required. The 'ward' team holds a daily teleconference (Lewis 2007). Such predictive modelling and care management by community matrons is now widespread in rural counties such as Cornwall, where 41 community matrons are based in GP surgeries (Lyndon 2007). These programmes can be supported by new software tools such as PARR (patients at risk of re-hospitalisation), developed by the Kings Fund, the Department of Health, New York University and Health Dialog. This gives a high rate of predictive accuracy and can be downloaded from www.kingsfund.org.uk/current_projects/predictive_risk/patients_at_risk. html.

The Pathways Service

The Pathways Service is a joint health and social care service, with a single assessment process using joint documentation, managed by Dudley Beacon and Castle Primary Care Trust and Dudley Social Services. A collaborative pathway of care for patients waiting for elective surgery is provided. A health and social care pre-assessment and discharge programme is carried out by a team of nurse and social work co-ordinators on each individual patient attached to GPs within the PCT area.

The objectives are to:

- reduce the incidence of pre-operative cancellations
- reduce the average length of stay
- prevent delayed hospital discharges when a patient is ready to go home
- reduce re-admission rates
- ensure patient satisfaction with hospital admission and discharge processes

One benefit is the introduction of a post of generic social care assistant jointly funded by the PCT and the Council who can carry out both health and social care assessments.

Joint working in Liverpool: two men at work

In 2004 and 2005, Liverpool City Council was strongly criticised for failing to properly administer nearly £50 million of Supporting People (SP) grant. Criticisms included a failure to monitor contracts and a tendency to act as a conduit for funding rather than as a commissioner and a regulator. By 2007, the service had been turned around, partly by focusing on instilling a value in all involved about impacting on outcomes for vulnerable adults, rather than just dispensing grant monies. A survey of SP providers conducted in May 2007 found that 58 per cent of respondents had engaged with new agencies to improve outcomes for service users, such as a GP practice visiting homeless service to assist service users in registering, and training agencies donating computers to temporary accommodation providers so service users could learn basic computing skills.

The improvement was partly driven by a strong working relationship between the Executive Director of Community Services in the City Council, Tony Hunter and the Chief Executive of the combined Liverpool PCT (from three previous PCTs for North, South and Central Liverpool), Derek Campbell. This partnership helped to drive up performance across a range of health and social care programmes, such as bringing delayed transfers of care down from several hundred to single figures. Co-terminosity between the two organisations was a key factor. The two men focused on helping each other, and recognising what mattered to each other, such as attaching social workers to hospital wards, much sought by the NHS but not at the time a priority for the City Council. They modelled mutual respect by never denigrating one another, and by expecting the same lack of negativity about their respective organisations from their staff. They both thought it vital to create an environment in which their respective staff groups could succeed and in which joint working was possible.

Liverpool Supporting People case study

Within Liverpool, Supporting People fund a refuge service for women experiencing domestic abuse from the black and minority ethnic community. A woman and her two children were referred to the service by the local police service. She had experienced domestic violence for a number of years and had involved the police for the first time. She was welcomed into the service and her support needs were identified leading to a support plan. With the support of the staff she was encouraged to engage with Merseyside Police and she took part in a resident self-help group, which built her confidence to pursue criminal charges against her abuser, who received a custodial sentence.

The refuge work in partnership with a local housing association and through this arrangement she secured her own tenancy for herself and her children. She received help to move into the tenancy and to furnish her new home, which in turn helped her to rebuild her life and confidence. She was successful in applying for a college course and her children settled into new schools. She has resettled well and is building links within her local community.

This approach could be usefully applied in the care of people with mental health problems, as 'one of the most pressing difficulties in compulsorily admitting a disturbed patient is getting all the necessary agents at the client's home at the correct time' (Bowers *et al.* 2003). This includes a psychiatrist, a community psychiatric nurse, an approved social worker, a GP and the patient's nearest relative or close friend(s), with the assessment co-ordinated by the approved social worker (ASW) in their care management role.

The growth in community care services in the last 30 years can also be illustrated by the way in which organisations have expanded, and in how the knowledge base for working with vulnerable adults has been put in place, all through partnership working. Little Women, a home care co-operative in Sunderland started by Margaret Elliott in 1976, has become Sunderland Home Care Associates, and has diversified into providing academic support for disabled university students. The Social Care Institute for Excellence (SCIE at www.scie.org.uk) and the National Institute for Clinical Excellence (NICE at www.nice.org.uk) have both published guidance, research and evaluation studies which promote best practice in the care and treatment of vulnerable adults. An example is the dementia care guide they have jointly produced, which for the first time means social care and NHS staff will work to the same guidance (NICE and SCIE 2006). This was much needed because three-quarters of people in care homes have dementia, but only 10 per cent of staff have adequate training, according to the Alzheimer's Society (Alzheimer's Society 2006). The knowledge base about service issues like ' dual diagnosis' – combined substance misuse and mental health problems, or combined mental health problems and a learning disability, is also advancing rapidly, particularly through partnership working between clinicians and researchers.

Domestic violence: partnership services

Sarah's story

'I was married to Gary for 15 years. For the first five years, I worshipped the ground that he walked on. However, that all changed when I had our son Billy. Gary started pouring all his love into Billy and blamed everything that went wrong in our lives onto me. It started with verbal abuse – small things at first but as the years went on the abuse grew worse. Gary was diagnosed as schizophrenic. He'd always had a drinking problem but the business failing had increased the amount he was drinking and the scale of abuse.' Sarah received beatings to her stomach and back, which she never let her family see. She said 'I tried to tell them what was happening to me but they were just as afraid of Gary because he would phone and threaten to harm Billy if they were involved. I tried to leave him several times but each time I had to leave Billy behind. I finally left him 18 months ago after he came home drunk and smashed all the house windows. I regret all the years I stayed with him but I can only look to the future.'

This is a tale of physical violence, but domestic violence is often accompanied by other forms of abuse such as sexual abuse, emotional abuse, financial abuse, psychological abuse, continual criticism and humiliation, movement monitoring, or threats to 'tell the authorities'. The pattern of domestic violence is similar to other social problems like drug abuse, in that prevention, stopping it through enforcement, and being able to give treatment through harm reduction programmes, are all important and all have to be made available simultaneously.

Domestic violence is a cross-cutting, complex and hard to reach social problem, ripe for partnership working programmes. The Croydon Family Justice Centre, the first in Europe of its kind, has 44 organisations working under one roof, including doctors, lawyers, police, probation, social workers, housing providers and benefits advisers. It was developed in partnership with the San Diego Family Justice Centre, an international centre of excellence for domestic violence services, and the New York Family Justice Centre. San Diego began co-ordinating services in 1975 and has seen a 75 per cent reduction in domestic homicides since then through a multi-agency partnership model, which seeks to integrate support and services for victims (ending homelessness, reducing incidents of abuse) with holding abusers accountable by co-ordinated monitoring. Croydon's centre developed out of various formal partnerships that developed between a number of US states and London, showing the value of twinning arrangements and knowledge exchanges, see Chapter 3 (Partnerships across countries and cultures).

In Cardiff, Multi-Agency Risk Assessment Conferences (MARACs) are held monthly and local agencies pool knowledge and information about high-risk cases. Repeat victimisation in Cardiff reduced from 30 per cent to less than 10 per cent in two years through this programme (Robinson 2004; Robinson and Tredidga 2007).

Transitions: joint working between children's and adult services

'Transition' is a key term in partnership working. Transition is a major feature of service users' lives: transitions between age groups, between countries, between homes, between cultures, between relationships, between jobs and between families. Staff supporting people who use services may themselves be in identical transitions: between jobs, between careers and sometimes between families and cultures too. This conveys a picture of transience on top of transition. Destabilisation, inconsistency, rapid change and temporary arrangements, are becoming a permanent feature of the social care world, even though continuity of care for vulnerable people is crucial.

A major transition to get right for service users is between childhood and young adulthood, when responsibility for care switches from one service to another. That transition is often managed poorly, with care packages, traditionally more generous in children's services, being instantly reduced

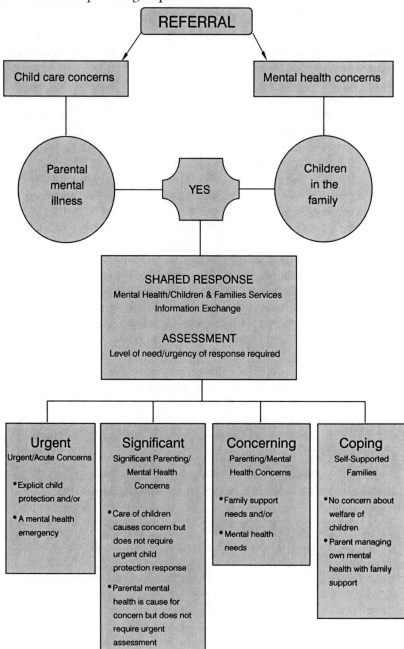

Figure 6.2 Camden Joint Service Protocol for Children and Families Affected by Mental Illness

Source: *Families That Have Alcohol and Mental Health Problems: A Template For Partnership Working, 2003*, Social Care Institute for Excellence, London

in adult services because of a different threshold and different budgetary limits. Families complain this is done with little if any notice, whereas ideally a joint assessment will be carried out at least two years in advance, with any reduction in a care package tapered over a period of time in agreement with the family concerned, including the young person or young adult. In fact the 'Transition Review for a child with Special Educational Needs should be the review following a disabled child's 14th birthday, when plans should start being formulated for their future and ... at each subsequent Annual Review, the Transition Plan should be considered and amendments made if necessary' (Jowitt and O'Loughlin 2005).

Given so much uncertainty over alternative plans and funding, clarity is important. 'How does the presence of children in families, for example, where a parent has mental health or alcohol abuse problems, change the eligibility criteria for both adult's and children's services? A protocol that includes arrangements for funding, joint or otherwise, needs to be part of the working relationship between the two services. The development of children's trusts and care trusts should also include clear requirements to account for these interface issues' (CSCI 2007).

Poor communication between children's and adult services has been identified as a major risk factor in serious case reviews following the death or serious injury of a child. These concerns continue. In a recent analysis of child deaths and serious injury, Brandon *et al.* found that:

> some of the children's parents were known to specialist adult services like substance misuse services or adult mental health services, but links were not made with children's social care ... As in previous studies of serious case reviews ... there was little evidence of shared expertise between specialist services like substance misuse services and domestic violence units with children's social care.
>
> (Brandon *et al.* 2008)

Some councils have been more pro-active than others. Kingston Council established a parent support worker post with a remit to work across children's and adult teams to promote parent support and joint working, including across agencies. In Mind the Gap, the Royal Borough of Kensington and Chelsea ran programmes to stop vulnerable people falling through the gaps between children's and adult services.

In conjunction with a pioneering specialist family court judge, Nick Crichton, Camden and Westminster Councils and local primary care trusts developed the first Family Drug and Alcohol Court in the country, just off Oxford Street in the West End of London. Modelled on similar courts in the USA, it aimed to combine criminal family and civil elements of a case in one court, and to ensure drug rehab services were available directly after a court appearance for a criminal offence.

In fairness to children, in fairness to their parents

Six children were removed from the care of two parents with learning disabilities following years of neglect, involving malnutrition and a lack of emotional attachment affecting all the children. By the time the local authority children's services team became aware of the situation, it was too late to reverse the abuse and damage faced by the children. Following a raft of expert assessments, some were placed in long-term foster care and some for adoption. However, the parents never received help from the council's learning disability service, as they did not meet the threshold for service provision, which was measured in terms of the severity of their adult disability. A combined threshold which took parenting ability as well as intrinsic learning disability into account would have easily led to priority eligibility for a joint service. A 'family plan', outlining the way in which the parents would be facilitated to develop the skills necessary to promote their children's development and to provide effective care and parenting for their children, would have been the right resource to jointly commission, months if not years before the crisis.

Working with drug-addicted parents and their children is a complex specialist area, especially as drugs are cheap and readily available throughout the UK, and easy for vulnerable people to slip into taking – 'You look really down. Try some of this'. The big issue in working with drug or alcohol misusers is to realise their main partnership is with the drugs or the booze – the substance becomes the most important family member for them. Children often prefer their drug-addicted parents not to go through rehab as it makes them more irritable and unstable, whereas drug workers role is to help their service user stay clean. Services have to align themselves in real time with drug misusers if rehab is to stand a chance of working. Above all, communication and understanding between the professionals working with children and the professionals working with adults has to be watertight.

An increasing number of families on social worker's caseloads feature the neglect of children as a result of one or both parents or carers having significant drug and alcohol problems, perhaps aligned with a mental health problem. Forrester and Harwin found that in 42 per cent of cases in four London boroughs between 2000 and 2005 where care proceedings were brought, the primary problem was a drug and/or alcohol problem, a much greater percentage than a generation before (Forrester and Harwin 2006). Additionally, a strong link between substance use and offending persists (Hagell 2002). Social workers have relatively little training in this area of work. Qualifying courses are slow to recognise the changing nature of caseloads and what students will imminently face as practitioners. Increasingly, academic tutors rely on a partnership with practice teachers when students are on placement to give them this knowledge. As one student told Bill Jordan:

> I trained as a joint practitioner in nursing and social work, and have now been qualified for just over a year. The first year has certainly been a learning curve. No amount of training really prepares a worker for the realities of fieldwork, or for fitting into the culture of an organisation.
>
> (Jordan 2006)

Single or combined approaches to multiple problems are also illustrated with the Single Asylum Fund, set up in 2003 to provide a single source of publicly funded legal advice and representation for asylum seekers.

Mature working between managers responsible for budgets can improve transition services. When communication is poor and cost shunting is suspected, a manager may go to a meeting, lose out, and come back and tell his or her staff: 'I bloody well told them', or, 'we're getting turned over', and staff can say back, 'Don't worry, at least you had a go'. Better management cultures ask middle managers with lead roles to resolve the issues logically and sensibly, by finding the best funding formula possible in the circumstances, rather than conducting management by sumo wrestling.

Inclusive practice: '*keeping the user in the team room*'

'Two years ago, you would not have got us to a meeting like this, let alone to be speaking at it' – the words of Julie and Lawrence, a couple who had both been through painful divorces and who now mentor other parents in that situation. Service users will be the future providers of many services.

Inclusive practice is a way of formalising a partnership working culture within agencies so it forms the basis for social care practice in individual cases. Social housing can be designed with toilets facing away from the south-east, so that tenants are not facing Mecca when they use them. A kitchen should have a powerful extractor fan built in as some Asian families prefer steam cooking which can give condensation problems. These are examples of culturally competent design and care based on universal service specifications which are sensitive to the needs of specific communities or groups without causing a problem to any other potential occupant. Using an electronic communication pad is crucial to be able to communicate at all with some people with learning disabilities. 'Is deodorant a luxury item?', is an issue for assessors of benefits. It does not sound like one, but for many people, deodorants are not a luxury item, but an essential toiletry which helps with cleanliness and self-esteem.

A swimming pool in Lewes, East Sussex, has a cubicle designed to accommodate wheelchair users, and fitness machinery for disabled people. Contrast this with 50 years ago, when people with disabilities were segregated from society in NHS homes and hospitals, and sometimes forced to eat their own vomit, not allowed visitors, forced to wear the underwear of their dead friends, and told they were about to die (*The Disabled Century*, BBC 2, 1999).

In father-inclusive practice – involving men remains one of the final frontiers in social care – a group of agencies got together to improve young fathers' experiences of maternity services. They were a national charity, a London teaching hospital and Sure Start. The national charity and the hospital built a strategic partnership which paved the way for the Sure Start worker to engage new fathers as they attended scans. He met with fathers-to-be, made contact with them for the future, and worked with midwives on necessary changes to the service' (Fathers Direct Toolkit, Card 9 on *Partnerships and Networks*).

The Chair of People First, the advocacy organisation for people with learning disabilities, travels from the North West of England for meetings in London despite having round the clock high support needs. Like many disabled people, he was told by professionals that he would never be able to achieve even a small measure of independence, but has proved them wrong. Inclusive practice supports people to realise their own dreams, rather than simply offering them a standard take it or leave it service from a fixed menu of provision. Pilot schemes to develop quality of life indicators for people with mental health problems, are involving patients in the development of satisfaction and outcome measures for services. The Centre for Policy on Ageing has been promoting the involvement of older people in housing planning decisions and design, and many programmes within the government's Partnerships with Older People programme, consisting of 29 local authority-led partnerships involving 298 organisations, 54 per cent from the voluntary sector, are producing positive outcomes through similar empowering approaches (University of Hertfordshire 2007).

As ever, the picture is a mixed and confusing one. Empowerment programmes in one sector can be contrasted with programmes where retrenchment is taking place, for example when local authorities take family centres back in house, away from voluntary organisations who were operating them via a contract, so the local authority has control over admissions.

The test of whether practice is inclusive is well expressed by children at Ealing's annual Powerful Voices conference, featuring presentations from over 100 young people from local schools. 'How will we know it's been a good day?' they asked, to be answered with, 'When we feel we've made a change' (Ealing Council 2006).

References

Alzheimer's Society, 2006, *Response to the GSCC Consultation on the Registration of Domiciliary and Residential Care Workers on their Social Care Register*, London: Alzheimer's Society.

Audit Commission, 2003, *Services for Disabled Children: A Review of Services for Disabled Children and their Families*, London: Audit Commission.

Barnardos, 2006, *Failed by the System: The Views of Young Care Leavers about their Educational Experiences*, London: Barnardos.

Borders Agency, 2008, *Better Outcomes: The Way Forward, Improving the Care of Unaccompanied Asylum Seeking Children*, London: Home Office.

Bowers, L., Clark, C. and Callaghan, P., 2003, 'Multi-disciplinary reflections on assessment for compulsory admission: the views of approved social workers, general practitioners, ambulance crews, police, community psychiatric nurses and psychiatrists', *British Journal of Social Work*, 33: 961–8.

Brandon, M., Belderson, P., Warren, C., Howe, D., Gardner, R., Dodsworth, J. and Black, J., 2008, *Analysing Child Deaths and Serious Injury Through Abuse and Neglect: What Can We Learn?* London: Department for Children, Schools and Families.

Bryan, H., Austin, B., Hailes, J., Parsons, C. and Stow, W., 2006, 'On track multi-agency projects in schools and communities: a special relationship', *Children and Society*, 20: 40–53.

Calder, M., 2004, *Assessment in Child Care: Identifying and Using Multi-Disciplinary Tools*, available from Martin Calder at Martinccalder@aol.com.

Calder, M. and Hackett, S., 2003, *Assessment in Child Care: Using and Developing Frameworks for Practice*, Lyme Regis: Russell House Publishing.

Cleaver, H., Walker, S. and Meadows, P., 2004, *Assessing Children's Circumstances: The Importance of the Assessment Framework*, London: Jessica Kingsley.

CSCI, 2008, *The State of Social Care in England*, London: Commission for Social Care Inspection.

CSCI, 2007, *Submission to the Green Paper, Care Matters*, London: Commission for Social Care Inspection.

Drogin, B., 2007, *Curveball*, London: Ebury Press.

DCSF, 2008, *Children's Trusts: Statutory Guidance on Inter-Agency Co-Operation to Improve Well-Being of Children, Young People and their Families*, London: Department for Children, School and Families.

Department of Health, 2007, *Commissioning a Brighter Future: Improving Access to Psychological Therapies*, London: Department of Health.

Eccles, A., 2008, 'Single shared assessment: the limits to 'quick fix' implementation', *Journal of Integrated Care*, 16(1): 22–30.

Fathers Direct, 2007, *Toolkit for Father-inclusive Practice*, London: Fathers Direct.

Forrester, D. and Harwin, J., 2006, 'Parental substance misuse and child care social work: findings from the first stage of a study of 100 families', *Child and Family Social Work*, 11(4): 325–35.

Hagell, A., 2002, *The Mental Health of Young Offenders – Bright Futures: Working With Vulnerable Young People*, London: Mental Health Foundation.

Harlow, E. and Shardlow, S., 2006, 'Challenges to the effective operation of core groups', *Child and Family Social Work*, 11: 65–72.

Jordan, B., 2006, Review of *'Well-Being: The Next Revolution in Children's Services'* in *Journal of Children's Services*, 1(1): 41–50.

Jowitt, M. and O'Loughlin, S., 2005, *Social Work with Children and Families*, Exeter: Learning Matters.

Katz, I. and Pinkerton, J., 2003, *Evaluating Family Support*, Chichester: John Wiley.

Kohli, R., 2005, 'The sound of silence: listening to what unaccompanied asylum children do and do not say', *British Journal of Social Work*, 1 of 15.

Kohli, R., 2006, 'The comfort of strangers: social work practice with unaccompanied asylum-seeking children and young people in the UK', *Child and Family Social Work*, 11: 1–10.

Lewis, G., 2007, 'Croydon Virtual Awards Scheme, a "ward without walls"', *The Guardian*, 28 November.

Lyndon, H., 2007, 'Community matrons – a conduit for integrated working?', *Journal of Integrated Care*, 15(6): 6–13.

Mental Health Act Commission, 2006, *11th Biennial Report*, London: Mental Health Act Commission.

Mental Health Act Commission, 2008, *12th Biennial Report*, London: Mental Health Act Commission.

National Institute for Clinical Excellence (NICE) and the Social Care Institute for excellence (SCIE), 2006, *Dementia: Supporting People with Dementia and their Carers in Health and Social Care*, London: NICE and SCIE (joint publication).

Polke, S., 2003, *History of Everything, Paintings and Drawings 1998–2003*, Dallas, TX: Dallas Museum of Art.

Robinson, A.L., 2004, *Domestic Violence MARACs for Very High Risk Victims in Cardiff, Wales: A Process and Outcome Evaluation*, Cardiff: Cardiff University.

Robinson, A.L. and Tredidga, J., 2007, 'The perceptions of high risk victims of domestic violence to a co-ordinated community response in Cardiff, Wales', *Violence against Women*, 13(11): 1130–48.

Social Exclusion Unit, 2008, *Think Family: Improving the Life Chances of Families at Risk*, London: Cabinet Office.

University of Hertfordshire, 2007, *National Evaluation of Partnerships for Older People's projects: interim Report on Progress*, London: Department of Health.

Whelan. R., 2004, *Robert Capa: The Definitive Collection*, London: Phaidon Press.

Young Voice, 2006, *Where is the Love: A Young Person's Guide to Understand, Prevent and Break Free of Dating Violence*, East Molesey: Young Voice.

7 Effective partnership working

Key messages

- The evidence base for partnership working is poor, but that is not the whole story
- The reasons why partnerships either succeed or fail are becoming clearer and are multi-factorial
- Proxy measures for partnership working can indicate a way forward, when it is too early for a formal evaluation
- Positive partnership outcomes can be more easily demonstrated in projects than in mainstream services

'The partnership is working very well but it hasn't delivered anything yet'.
(quote from an energy industry consultant,
in Huxham and Vangen 2005)

'If a lot of cures are suggested for a disease, it means the disease is incurable'.

(Anton Chekhov, *The Cherry Orchard*)

Measuring effectiveness: the challenges

The evidence base for success is missing, or ambiguous

As we have seen in Chapter 1, partnerships are usually set up to solve problems beyond the ability of a single person or organisation to influence. However, that is no guarantee of success. As Frost points out, the evidence base for partnership working models is problematic – 'while the task of reviewing the research, say on child placement, would provide relatively clear limits, this is not the case with partnership working. The literature is diffuse' (Frost 2005). This echoes earlier findings, suggesting that the time-scale to fully implement a partnership working model is much longer than first realised: 'the consensus among researchers is that partnership arrangements consume a huge amount of time, energy and resources to create relatively limited outcomes and outputs' (Percy-Smith 2006). Much that is said about partnership working is based on beliefs rather than facts, and strongly-held beliefs are hard to change or mediate.

A literature search on health and social care partnerships published in the UK since 1997 showed little evidence of better outcomes for service users (Dowling *et al.* 2004). Similar pessimistic conclusions have been reached about a range of high-profile programmes, like Sure Start (Belsky *et al.* 2007). Optimistic evaluations tend to emphasise future prospects more than current achievements.

Between health and social care, 'research tends to support the notion that the two professions are still in an evolving, indeterminate relationship' (Pierson 2008). A key issue is that social care practitioners and managers frequently have to take action in situations when they know both outcomes and value for money will be poor. The rhetoric of perpetual improvement and effectiveness can be contrasted with the day to day reality when social care professionals are hastily assembling, often in a crisis, imperfect support or protection arrangements for people, that are 'just about good enough'. The same holds true for other professions. When asked why they sentence offenders to a prison sentence, when they often know it won't work, judges and magistrates say they do not know what else to do – they are not being given positive alternatives. Social care is similar. Having said that, 'just about good enough' can be the difference between life and death. Patching a situation up can give valuable breathing space to all involved.

Even if nothing much changes as a result of a social care intervention, the intervention might still be justifiably classified as successful. As the child-care expert and pioneer Barbara Kahan used to say, institutional care can be both positive and negative, and residential care has pluses and minuses for individual service users – it is neither all good, nor is it always bad. A risk in the current rush towards 'personalisation' and personal budgets for service users, is that residential care is becoming forgotten again, including good residential care. Some service users may be prematurely pushed into holding a personal budget they cannot manage. In providing services, and in evaluating social care's achievements and performance, it is important to be neither half-full nor half-empty, nor to focus on one policy or service provision to the exclusion of all others.

Successful partnerships are also impossible to guarantee because the number of factors to predict or control when two or more organisations collaborate increases through a multiplier effect. According to David Bell, the Permanent Secretary in the Department of Children, Schools and Families, 'It is very significant that the (new) Public Service Agreements (PSAs) exemplify cross-government ambitions. That is going to be tough because our experience of the last PSA round is that the shared PSAs (i.e. shared between several different government departments) were sometimes

Finding a cure for scurvy: 'it takes time to discover what works'

A cure for scurvy was only finally made available to all seafarers in the mid-nineteenth century, following the pioneering work of a surgeon, James Lind: a mariner, Captain Cook; and a physician, Gilbert Blane, over the course of a hundred years from Lind through to Blane (Bown 2003). Scurvy had plagued ships for several hundred years before that, often killing more than half of every crew. Identifying the need for lemon juice and fresh vegetables to ensure sailors had sufficient Vitamin C hardly sounds radical thinking now, but it took hundreds of years to realise both the exact nature of the problem, and the cure.

harder to achieve' (Bell 2007). That theme, of 'difficult but desirable' has been echoed and reinforced throughout this book.

Partnership working is an 'empirical minefield' (Glendinning *et al.* 2002). Proxy outcomes such as partnership processes often demonstrate more success than directly measurable improved outcomes for people who use services. Outcomes are hard to measure, 'loose talk about outcomes can be misleading' (Petch 2007), and 'empirical studies ... do not provide clear answers (Scott *et al.* 2003), despite the hotch-potch of solutions offered in partnership cookbooks. Partnerships tend to be new services or organisations, and they take time to set up, bed in, establish a new infrastructure and deliver results. Occasional public, political and press impatience with this is illustrated in the coverage of the London 2012 Olympic Games development programme in east London. Within a few months of the Olympic Delivery Authority starting up, concerns were being expressed about a lack of progress, whereas visible progress is unlikely until much closer to 2011. The first few years of any major project or partnership are invisible developmental stages, but that does not mean the partnership is ineffective. What matters is that continuous progress is made through a clear project plan with an accurate timeline, a little like boring a hole under a river for a road or rail tunnel: suddenly, years after boring starts, the cutting machine breaks through on the other side.

So, it takes time for the impact and effectiveness of a new public policy to be assessed, and then for a best practice model to be widely disseminated.

Allowing time for a partnership to blossom does not mean persevering with an obviously ineffective one. A more 'agile' approach to government means that if a programme does fail to deliver, its funding should be stopped and rapidly re-directed (Filkin 2007).

Re-framing failure, if not as success, as acceptable progress

Similarly, building up a contacts list, a knowledge base and intelligence partnerships took the CIA and MI6 years before they could start to run safe operations. Many positive developments may, as Amanda Edwards suggests, 'be re-cast as failure, rather than progress or limited achievement', because unless dramatic progress can be seen and measured within an unrealistically short time-scale, there is a tendency to assume it will never be made. This quick fix mentality may undermine long-term progress, which is nurtured through stability, not turbulence (Edwards 2007).

Benefits realisation from partnership working – compared to the investment made and the costs over time – is hard to quantify, especially as benefits may not be realised for several years, and the organisations involved may suffer short-term losses en route. Applying a public value test for additionality or added value is complicated (Hudson and Hardy 2002). The government-commissioned Atkinson Review, into the measurement of outputs and productivity across government services found that personal social services were too difficult to measure coherently, in that the contribution of informal carers to good outcomes for vulnerable people was not included in any measure of state support, and 'for certain individuals, the increment to welfare may be simply the prevention of further or faster decline than might otherwise have occurred' (Atkinson 2005).

No way back

Although it can't be demonstrated that partnership working in itself is always successful, it does not follow it should be abandoned. It is more sensible to take steps to increase its likely effectiveness in the future. A return to silo-based working, even if it were possible, is a recipe for returning to practices already widely condemned as ineffective. A difficulty with the future should not precipitate a voyage back into the past. Several innovative social care developments , such as 'In My Shoes', an interactive computer programme to promote effective communication about sensitive issues with young children, vulnerable children and vulnerable adults, took ten years to develop. The Chairman of Families Need Fathers, John Baker, told me it would take a generation to secure equal rights for fathers, not the few months that hard-line activists sought. Just as lack of short-term progress disillusions some, it is hard for anyone to know exactly what to do in the short-term if a change process will take as long as a generation, although as the French Marshal Lyautey said to his gardner, when told a particular tree he liked would take one hundred years to grow to maturity, 'there is no time to lose, plant it this afternoon'.

Partnership working outcomes

Getting the baseline right

The key to measuring effectiveness is to get the baseline right, whether for an individual service user, or a service as a whole, as it has been for league tables with schools. An additional point to bear in mind is that the consequence of social care partnerships is that added value may come from other, indirect support services available to service users, following discussions with social care staff and advice received, for example through housing officers, volunteers, or carers. Measured services are not the only ones being provided or received.

Many partnership developments are self-evidently an improvement on what was in place before. The Partnership Primary Care Centre in Islington is a purpose-built centre, supporting a range of services including the local multi-disciplinary long-term conditions team. It was previously a run-down GP practice. By any standards, the partnership development represents an improvement – in the working environment for professionals, in the training facilities which enhance the learning of many staff groups who use them, and in the contribution to the regeneration of the local area made by the new building. Partnership outcomes are often subtle and invisible, yet legion. A common sense set of measurements will often highlight a set of specific local improvements beyond the analytical reach of inspectors, auditors and researchers. The long-term partnership between the NSPCC and Sport England will ensure that all sports organisations are accredited by the NSPCC as having appropriate child protection measures in place by 2009, working within the framework of the National Standards for Safeguarding Children in Sport. This partnership, like many thousands of others, will bring indisputable indirect benefits.

Proxy measures

The difficulty in measuring or establishing effectiveness is illustrated by the lack of an accepted model for partnership working or a nationally agreed set of outcome-based performance indicators. Proxy measures have to be used instead, to show indirect benefit. For example, an increase in the number of young adults with physical disabilities provided with personalised independent living services is likely to be a sign of a strong partnership between the commissioning organisation and the people who use its services. Good structures and local enabling protocols are likely to lead to better outcomes. Local Criminal Justice Boards have helped to transform crown prosecutor behaviour and attitude by engaging them in considering the impact of their own actions on sanctioned detection rates. Most studies of partnership services give a strong clue or steer about what to do to increase the chances of successful outcomes. For example, whilst the evaluations of Sure Start

First, find out who the partnership is with, then whether it is effective

In my first week as an unqualified social worker in the Rhondda Valley, in 1975, I was allocated the case of a 15-year-old boy in care, Robert, who had run away from countless placements but who was now settled in an adult ward of the local psychiatric hospital. The psychiatrist kept discharging him, and he kept returning. I had no advice from my supervisor, so the reflective supervision partnership, so important when you start out as a social worker, was ineffective. The day after I met him, having been refused re-entry for the umpteenth time, he jumped out of a high window at the hospital and killed himself. I was outraged, and wanted to speak out about what I saw as negligence on the part of the psychiatrist. I felt I had a working partnership with the boy's family and much less than this with my own department. The Director of Social Services threatened me with the sack if I spoke out. I felt that senior staff across agencies were in a collusive partnership to suppress the truth coming out – I may have been right, I may have been wrong. It is hard to know when you're young and starting out. The boy's parents and I corresponded for a while, but eventually we lost touch. The partnerships on the ground, within the family and between the family and professionals, left all concerned feeling a sense of hopelessness and 360 degree betrayal.

In July 2007, 32 years later, in a parliamentary answer, the English Health Under Secretary, Ivan Lewis, said that projects which help to eliminate the inappropriate use of adult psychiatric wards for children and young people will get preference in future NHS mental health funding decisions. Spending on child and adolescent mental health services (CAMHS) is now increasing year on year, offering some hope for the future. Many young people I have worked with, who had apparent severe behaviour problems, in fact had unrecognised (at the time) mental health problems, which went untreated in the crucial early years.

Psychiatric units as a place of refuge continue to turn people in need away. Andrew Howlett pleaded with staff at the Maudsley Hospital, where he had been treated for two months, to stay. Five months later, he said he felt trapped in his flat' and set out to 'do anybody'. 'Anybody' was his neighbour, Michael Galloway, who Howlett attacked and killed with multiple stab wounds. Howlett was sentenced to be detained in a secure mental hospital (BBC News, 9 November 2006). In March 2008, it was reported that NHS London admitted that the statutory review that should have taken place into Howlett's care, had not been (BBC News, 4 March 2008).

Ever since the de-institutionalisation movement of the 1970s (Scull 1977), the numbers of residential and nursing care beds for vulnerable adults has been reducing, to the point where the in-patient population is now distilled to people in acute psychotic states. Many more people with complex needs are being looked after through partnership working between community learning disability services, community mental health services, housing management services, primary care services and from time to time more specialist services. This has meant liberation for some, and a new form of abandonment for others.

are cautious about what it can achieve, Allnock *et al.* (2006) identified a framework for effective partnership working, based on the following findings and observations:

- building new partnerships takes time
- there is likely to be a hierarchy of engagement, as, at any one time, different agencies will have different priorities
- even if there is a dearth of inherited positive inter-agency linkages, proactive networking by key stakeholders, especially at higher management levels, can help make good the deficits
- 'targets' need to be relevant across agencies: if so they can actually help; if not, they are a major impediment to partnership
- in particular targets for preventive work are crucial; they need to apply *across disciplines*, not, as is currently the situation, to exclude statutory social work
- chief executives are in a position to maximise the likelihood of inter-agency collaboration if their commitment can be clearly seen by their workforce
- it is essential that different professional groups respect and acknowledge the value of 'others' in order to establish trust about information sharing and appropriate referrals.

So what can we say about outcomes?

In terms of measurable outcomes as a result of statutory partnerships, here are just a few.

Barnsley and other places

The benefits of partnership working, initially through the Barnsley Health Action Zone and more recently through inter-agency programmes led by Barnsley PCT, led directly to improved public health outcomes such as an increase in life expectancy for men in the most health disadvantaged areas in Barnsley of 3.3 years between 1997/99 and 2004/06. In the same time period, the gap in life expectancy between the most health disadvantaged areas and the average narrowed from 4.1 years to 2.5 years.

And as well as this:

- Brighton and Hove reduced the number of rough sleepers in the town from 66 in 2001 to 12 in 2006.
- Street homelessness in London reduced from 5,000 to 500 in the decade from 1997 to 2007, partly due to the Rough Sleepers Initiative, a central-government driven partnership programme. Rough sleepers were also supported by some pioneering local partnership services such

as the Cardiff City Centre Rough Sleepers Team, who provided a range of mobile outreach services from a converted double decker bus.

- A partnership between Prudential 4 Youth and Crime Concern led to a 16 per cent reduction in the theft of mobile phones through the Wolverhampton Mander Centre project; a 21.6 per cent reduction in insurance claims as a result of malicious damage through the Manchester Arndale project; and a 70 per cent reduction in youth nuisance through the Washington Galleries project between 2000 and 2005.

The evaluation of the Positive Activities for Young People (PAYP) programme concluded youth activities can deliver positive outcomes in relation to crime health and education for 84 per cent of those at risk of social exclusion. The TXT Zone project in West Orchards Shopping Centre, Coventry, allows members of the public to text a security team if they feel unsafe, leading to flash patrols and 74 per cent of customers saying they feel safer. The London Borough of Barking and Dagenham went from satisfying local people least of all the 33 London boroughs in 2004, to satisfying them most in 2006, as a result of a sustained focus on their partnership with local residents.

In fact, most local areas and service providers can point to success stories, even if outcome measures are lacking. Many new developments should lead to long-term gains. As Neil Hunter, Joint General Manager of Glasgow Addiction Services (GAS), said:

> The number of people receiving addiction services has doubled in 4 years, because we have brought the organisations together. We have not only doubled our resources but we have created efficiencies in the system. What we have now is a template for the future
>
> ('No pain, no gain', *The Guardian* Society supplement, 1 November 2006)

Social care outcomes are harder to measure than outcomes for services like education, in which pupils who are the same age follow a national curriculum and sit standard tests at defined points in their education. Comparing test results with previous scores provides a sound basis for calculating the value added by a school and is a reliable way to measure progress. Once the system is in place, it can be contextualised to take into account variables such as social disadvantage.

By contrast, social care services are highly individualised and social care services do not stand alone – other services like health and education also have an impact on the well-being of a person using services, so it is hard to calculate the added value or worth of each service separately. What can be measured, along with proxy outcomes, are the inputs that are likely to make a contribution to better outcomes: these include the allocation for a period of time of a skilled and experienced caseworker who becomes actively engaged with a service user or their family; and a good multi-agency assessment and care plan which is agreed with the service user and implemented.

The Commission for Social Care's (CSCI) proposed new outcomes framework for the performance assessment of adult social care (2006), was peppered with references to the importance of joint working. A key line of assessment 1 (out of nine), which measures improvement in health and well-being, only gives an excellent rating (score of 4) if there is 'well-developed and consistent' joint working with health partners and 'other relevant agencies'. Conversely an inadequate rating (score of 1) will be partly due to 'limited joint working', with work 'poorly co-ordinated and not built on shared objectives'. A key line of assessment 6, which measures economic well-being, only gives an excellent rating if 'the partnership between the local authority, the Learning and Skills Council, and the business sector is constructive and the very high quality of collaboration between partners leads to very effective guidance to all groups of people, including vulnerable and minority ethnic groups, and those with complex needs'. An inadequate rating follows on from the partnership 'not being well established, with collaboration between partners leading to poor advice and guidance to all people'. Inspection and auditing frameworks are powerful levers to control organisational priorities, and all current inspection frameworks stipulate a high level of partnership working.

Partnership toolkits

Evaluation of partnership working and integrated care can consider different aspects of integration, such as integration functioning, integration synergy and integration effectiveness (Lasker *et al.* 2001). However, there are limits to what can be measured, and 'it seems impossible to create a comprehensive measurement model which takes fully into account the multi-dimensional context of integrated care' (Ahgren 2007). This does not mean evaluation is futile, rather that members of a partnership should select the tools they feel most comfortable using, and which can be applied to their own partnership easily with minimal adaptation.

Toolkits to evaluate partnership working abound, many of them useful to practitioners and analysts. The best examples are:

• The Nuffield Institute's Partnership Assessment Tool (Nuffield Institute 2000) described six principles for effectiveness including ownership, monitoring partnership agreements, and learning from experience. The Strategic Partnering Taskforce, set up by the Office of the Deputy Prime Minister in England, considered how this might be applied to strategic partnerships, and produced a self-assessment toolkit for partners, including a rapid partnership profile scoring system to assess progress (Hardy *et al.* 2003).

- Research in Practice has developed an action pack and range of tools to audit team or partnership working across the four domains of partnership working of Anning *et al.* (2006):
  1 structural (systems and management)
  2 ideological frameworks (sharing skills and beliefs)
  3 procedural influences (developing new processes)
  4 inter-professional learning through role change (Garrett and Lodge 2008).
- The Partnership Outcomes Evaluation Toolkit (POET) is a resource developed by the Health Services Management Centre (HSMC) as a web-based resource focusing on both the process and outcomes of partnership working.
- Q Learning have developed a Partnership Health Check (www. partnershiphealthcheck.com) and a partnership checklist for self-evaluation and self-assessment.
- Thorlby and Hutchinson's guide to partnership working, produced for The New Opportunities Fund, draws on established good practice and research and includes a number of case studies (New Opportunities Fund 2002).
- The National Outcomes Framework for Community Care in Scotland and the UDSET (User-defined Service Evaluation Toolkit) is being piloted in eight health and social care partnerships throughout Scotland, and is being evaluated using service user researchers (Miller *et al.* 2008). Initially it proved difficult to isolate the effects of partnership working. Partnerships were asked to gather data on the following service user outcomes:
  - percentage of community care service users feeling safe
  - percentage of users of community care services and carers satisfied with their involvement in their health and social care packages
  - percentage of users of community care services reporting satisfaction with the opportunities provided for meaningful interaction
  - percentage of carers feeling supported and capable of continuing in their role as carer.
- Smith and Beazley's Wheel of Involvement (2000) focuses on partnership outcomes.
- Methodologies such as Experian's mosaic classification system, which identifies the make-up and mix of neighbourhoods, and the Organisational Culture Inventory and Nursing Unit Cultural Assessment tool, can be extended to the analysis of partnerships.
- The Picker Institute aims to bring the patient perspective on judging whether user-defined outcomes are being achieved, using survey methods.
- The National Council of Voluntary Organisations proposed a way of arriving at the outcome value, financial value, equity value, activity value and excellence value of a voluntary sector project or service (Bolton 2002).

- The Audit Commmission has an ' effective partnership working test' with 28 questions (www.auditcommission.gov.uk) (Audit Commission, 1998).
- Outcome-based evaluation (OBE) programmes (Fagan *et al.* 2007) – measuring outcomes is now the norm, despite its difficulty: NCH and Barclays Bank evaluate their Financial Futures project for young people using the London Benchmarking model, so that they can show the difference they make to young people in ways such as their bank accounts staying in the black and tenancies maintained.
- Markwell has brought together a useful guide to partnership working resources (Markwell 2003).
- West and Markiewicz (2006) developed an effective partnership working inventory, aiming to measure the seven dimensions of effective partnership working (see Figure 7.1).

Toolkits do not have to be unduly complicated. For example, the degree of partnership working between a social care agency and its BME service users and staff can be assessed by an independent researcher asking the right questions in a simple survey. The will to ask the right questions and act on the answers matters as much as excessive reliance on toolkits.

Evaluations are now routinely being shared with people who use services. In April 2008, the Court of Appeal ruled that the National Institute of

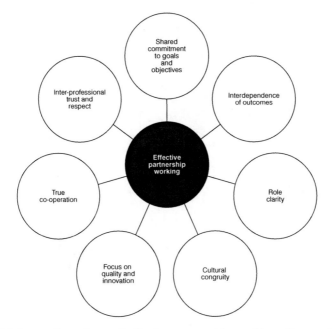

Figure 7.1 Seven dimensions of effective partnership working (Source: West and Markewicz 2006)

Partnership Self-Assessment Tool

Assessment Question	Guidance notes	Assessment Decision Score			Action! To improve the effectiveness of the partnership
Section A: Foundations					
A1 Does the partnership have SMART objectives shared by all its partners? (SMART = Specific, Measurable, Achievable, Results Focused, & Time Limited).	Strategic objectives should be clear and all partners should agree on them. Are they SMART? It may be useful to think that if someone actually observed the partnership operate would they be able to identify what it was trying to achieve? Equally the partnership's objectives should be consistent with other relevant strategic plans & priorities.	NO (1) action is required ☐	YES (2) but could be improved ☐	YES (3) working effectively ☐	
A2 Is the partnership accountable to anyone? (Does it link or report to any other partnership groups?)	The partnership should have a clear line of accountability within the health and social care structures in Leeds. It may be accountable to an individual or another partnership group such as the Health Inequalities and Modernisation Board. It should also link where appropriate to other partnership groups to avoid duplication.	NO (1) action is required ☐	YES (2) but could be improved ☐	YES (3) working effectively ☐	
A3 Does the partnership make decisions?	The partnership may have a valid role as a networking forum. However, it should have a responsibility for completing a task, or setting priorities to be effective and not be regarded as a 'talking shop'. In terms of making decisions over resources is it important to define exactly what (if any) resources are influenced or controlled by the partnership.	NO (1) action is required ☐	YES (2) but could be improved ☐	YES (3) working effectively ☐	
A4 Are the costs of the partnership known and weighed up against the benefits?	Need to include the costs of organising and attending meetings & progressing work between meetings. Benefits could be considered in terms of the costs of not working in partnership i.e. what would happen if the partnership did not exist?	NO (1) action is required ☐	YES (2) but could be improved ☐	YES (3) working effectively ☐	

Partnership Self-Assessment Tool

Assessment Question	Guidance notes	Assessment Decision Score			Action! To improve the effectiveness of the partnership

Section B: The Partners

Assessment Question	Guidance notes	NO (1) action is required	YES (2) but could be improved	YES (3) working effectively	Action!
B1 Does the partnership take into account the different cultures of partners?	Different individual and organisational cultures should be recognised & worked with in a positive way. Shared training and time spent to understand each partner's organisation, culture and practices is invaluable and will reduce the opportunity for conflict. E.g. it is important that local authority colleagues understand the NHS culture is centrally driven and that NHS colleagues appreciate the political agenda driving the local authority.	☐	☐	☐	
B2 Is there commitment to the partnership at an appropriate senior level?	Without suitable commitment the partnership is likely to lack the ability to achieve its stated objectives. Partners may need to be able to make certain decisions on behalf of their organisations. Try to establish why senior level support is not there and give support to organisations trying to obtain commitment.	☐	☐	☐	
B3 Does the partnership have the necessary skills to fulfil its objectives?	There should be a learning culture within the partnership which allows partners to gain new knowledge & skills. Training and secondments may be useful. Alternatively other partners with the desired knowledge & skills may need to be brought in.	☐	☐	☐	
B4 Is there an appropriate balance of power in the partnership?	Is there is a hierarchy? e.g. does the statutory sector have a higher status & influence than the voluntary sector. If some partners dominate then others may become less active and lose interest. Power and responsibility need to be shared. This may require some partners to give some up and others to take more on.	☐	☐	☐	

Figure 7.2 Partnership Assessment toolkit

Partnership Self-Assessment Tool

Assessment Question	Guidance notes	Assessment Decision Score			Action! To improve the effectiveness of the partnership
Section C: Communication and Involvement					
C1 Are the partnership meetings effective?	Consider factors like: Attendance levels. Is the venue/room layout suitable? Do all partners actively participate? Do you need to set some ground rules about the use of jargon, keeping to time etc? Meetings may not always be appropriate, workshops or less formal events could also be used.	NO (1) action is required	YES (2) but could be improved	YES (3) working effectively	
C2 Is there good communication within the partnership?	Documentation such as minutes could be in more friendly formats e.g. key action points/newsletter. Is enough use made of e mail? How do partners communicate outside meetings? There may be a reliance on informal networks which exclude some partners.	NO (1) action is required	YES (2) but could be improved	YES (3) working effectively	
C3 Is information about the work and achievements of the partnership communicated to people outside it?	It is important that the partnership communicates with key stakeholders. May be appropriate to hold an annual stakeholder event, publish a newsletter, or make information available on the web. Such methods could be used to gain feedback to inform the work of the partnership.	NO (1) action is required	YES (2) but could be improved	YES (3) working effectively	
C4 Is there effective user, carer or public involvement?	How much do they contribute? What support is in place to ensure effective representation e.g. could they have a "buddy" within the partnership. (Please refer to the User and Carer Involvement Toolkit available from the Health Action Zone team 0113 305 9581)	NO (1) action is required	YES (2) but could be improved	YES (3) working effectively	

Partnership Self-Assessment Tool

Section D: Measuring and reviewing Success

Assessment Question	Guidance notes	Assessment Decision Score			Action! To improve the effectiveness of the partnership
		NO (1) action is required	YES (2) but could be improved	YES (3) working effectively	
D1 Has the partnership set clear performance targets?	The partnership should have arrangements to measure the impact of its work. Outcomes may consist of numerical and other performance indicators. They should be designed to clearly demonstrate when an objective has been achieved.	NO (1) action is required	YES (2) but could be improved	YES (3) working effectively	
D2 Is progress towards targets actively monitored and reported?	Progress against performance indicators should be monitored. Regular reports on progress should be given to partners e.g. quarterly.	NO (1) action is required	YES (2) but could be improved	YES (3) working effectively	
D3 Is there an end point when the partnerships work is likely to be complete?	Some partnerships are created to undertake a specific task but still continue to operate once the task is complete. It is important to discontinue a partnership if it no longer has a clear purpose. An exit strategy may need to be considered for handing over the work.	NO (1) action is required	YES (2) but could be improved	YES (3) working effectively	
D4 Are the partnership arrangements regularly reviewed?	Strategic objectives, terms of reference and membership should be regularly reviewed and revised accordingly. Reviews should take into account both process and task related issues.	NO (1) action is required	YES (2) but could be improved	YES (3) working effectively	
Date of Assessment		TOTAL SCORE			Next Assessment due

Figure 7.2 Partnership Assessment toolkit (continued)

Health and Clinical Excellence (NICE) must share with patients and their representatives the economic model it uses as the basis for its decisions about whether a particular new drug on the market represents value for money to the NHS. The basis for all social care decision making and the appraisals of how decisions about funding allocations or practice models are made, should in this day and age be publicly available, just as the basis for decision making in cases should be available in its entirety to the person using the service.

Why do some partnerships succeed?

Any description of what works well and not so well begs the question of the eyes being looked through, in particular whether the outlook is an optimistic or a pessimistic one (Hudson 2002). Quinney has challenged academics to test out more positive hypotheses (Quinney 2006). Many services and organisations are both good and bad. When they are rated as excellent, that will conceal pockets of poor practice, just as a negative rating will conceal pockets of excellence. In describing Liverpool as the European City of Culture in 2008, commentators veered between highlighting the major events taking place, and the debts the City Council would still be paying off for years to come. In reality, the level of debt will be small for a city with a budget the size of Liverpool's, and the real success of City of Culture status will lie in the extra regeneration generated from the raised profile and the sustainability of the programmes into the long-term cultural life of the city. That measurement will probably not be possible much before 2015.

Partnership between Maltby BEST and Rotherham Young Minds

Maltby BEST (Behaviour Education and Support team) is a co-located fully integrated multi-agency team of professionals drawn from health, education and the voluntary sector. Rotherham Young Minds service employs four staff to work within the BEST team, which also has four other mental health workers and two trainer/consultants. The team has developed an anti-bullying pathway, used in secondary schools throughout Rotherham. Whilst 53 per cent of students reported having being bullied recently before the project started, 71 per cent reported not being bullied or being bullied less at exit from the project.

An emphasis is put on finding individual children a way a manageable way of dealing with the pressures on them, and developing training packages for professionals, including financing a borough-wide 'Miss Dorothy' package, which provides a resource to be used within the school curriculum across all Key Stages.

Despite the methodological difficulties, it is clear that successful and sustainable partnerships are happening in many places, and equally obvious that they're not happening everywhere. Glendinning *et al.* (2000) have suggested a number of factors that may support effective partnerships:

- a history of collaborative working
- co-terminous boundaries
- commitment from the senior managers in all partner agencies
- committed resource and project management capacity.

If this is starting to sounds repetitive, it is because most researchers make the same points and come to similar conclusions about partnership working.

Partnerships usually work well in a crisis

Following a disaster, like the fire at Kings Cross in 1987, the London Underground bombings in 2005, flooding in the West Country in 2007 and mass temporary evacuations of local people from their homes following bomb scares, the emergency services invariably work well together, including social care staff who provide a range of immediate and follow-up services like counselling. Social care staff are committed and will come out at any time of the day and night when asked.

In the inquiry into the murders of five young prostitutes in Ipswich in 2006, over 500 officers from 36 police forces were involved, mostly specialists. Suffolk County Council's social exclusion team supported Ipswich prostitutes to stay off the street by paying for drug rehab services. The police offered an amnesty from scrutiny of sex work whilst the killer, the subsequently convicted Steve Wright, remained at large. The partnership approach carried on after Wright's arrest, in an attempt to influence and change the lifestyles of the women concerned.

Why do some partnerships fail?

Elitism or perceived elitism

Smaller partners can feel excluded by bigger partners, causing resentment, or an inner elite can be mistrusted by a wider group of partners. Spain, Poland and the new smaller states in the European Union often resent France, Germany and Britain for holding restricted meetings between themselves leading to suspicion they are 'stitching up' the agenda. Political history is littered with concerns about elitism at all levels. The US/UK invasion of Iraq in 2003 was widely held to be the product of a secret deal between George Bush and Tony Blair. The Sykes–Picot agreement in 1916, (a secret Anglo-French deal, planned to parcel up the Middle East, but which never came off as the Russians, who were in on the secret, publicised it when Lenin came to power in 1917) has fuelled suspicion of Western intentions ever since. Suspicion or evidence of deceit, particularly where resources or decision-making are concerned, undermines the chances of partnership working being effective.

Many people within social care approach partnerships with caution, fearing the profession 'will be consigned to junior partner status in some partnerships, as social care is often "the dog that didn't bark"' (Jordan and Jordan 2000). Or else a particular individual or agency, who feels excluded or marginalised, will say to themselves, 'why wasn't I mentioned?' in a roll call of thanks about starting a partnership up, which concentrates on the higher profile names and players. Exclusion may be real, not just perceived – 'The co-ordinator of a health promotion partnership was unable to name quickly all the partners involved in the partnership even though they are well defined, relatively small in number and listed on partnership note paper' (Huxham and Vangen 2005).

An inability to transcend hierarchical thinking inhibits successful partnerships. 'The concept of a hierarchy of professions differentiated by full and semi-professional status has a particular relevance for health and social care professions which have contrasting histories and contrasting contemporary circumstances on such matters as length of training, legal registration and the right to practice. Joint work may be more difficult where there are perceived status differentials between team members (Carrier and Kendall 1995).

In a CSCI report into older peoples services in Northumberland – the first care trust set up to commission health and social care services – the trust was criticised for failing to give social care sufficient priority. The inspection, carried out in 2005, found no benefit to social care since the trust was set up in 2002. Inspectors found managers overstretched and focusing on health priorities rather than social care. Social care had little visibility in board meetings and performance and care management systems were weak. The risk of social care, or any smaller partner, not being given equal status inside new joint organisations, is a significant threat to the development of a successful partnership culture (see Chapter 5).

Pressure of the internal agenda: partnership overload and fatigue

In 2007, the Cabinet Secretary, Gus O'Donnell, asked departmental permanent secretaries to let him know the percentage of their time they spent working within their departments, across Whitehall and with outside organisations. They said the ratio was 100:0:0. When told this was the wrong answer, and that they needed to work harder both across Whitehall and externally, they replied the ratio was 100:15:10! All a long time after Harold Macmillan, the British Prime Minister from 1957 to 1963, talking informally to a friend of mine in 1962, said, 'this job is getting far too busy. I now only get time to read two novels a week'.

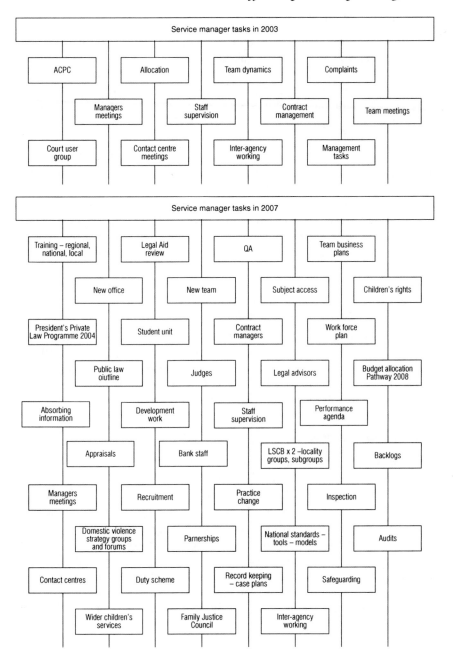

Figure 7.3 Service manager timeline 2003–07

Inexorably increasing workloads

Figure 7.3 shows the huge increase in the range and volume of tasks demanded of service managers in Cafcass, the national organisation representing the interests of children and young people in family court cases in England. It shows a three-fold increase in demands between 2004 and 2007. Every task is important but each one adds to the bureaucratic burden, which often feels unmanageable. The more varied the work, the higher the risks. As a social worker operating across several projects commented, 'I find it hard to juggle the three projects. You're asking me to spread myself thinly on the ground and not do anything properly' (Moran *et al.* 2007). The issues are similar for managers and practitioners. When I was a director of many operational services in a London Borough, including being Director of Housing, Social Services, Revenues and Benefits, Leisure and Culture, with the aim of creating joined-up government, I ended up being a classic Jack of all trades and master of none – changing a structure is not in itself an integrating mechanism.

Many new policy and practice trends like personalisation (see Chapter 2) bring with them demands – as a professional, you have to get to know everyone, which takes time you don't have.

It is a truism that people are working harder, whatever their job. Hard work and long hours is now an intrinsic part of UK culture, more so than in most other countries. Most organisations are having to concentrate on their 'core business' to make sure basic services continue to be provided day in, day out. Faced with this, partnership working can seem a luxury.

Essential partnerships only

The implication of this 'back to basics' or 'stay with the basics' reality of life in social care, is to restrict the number of partnerships at any one time to those that can demonstrate clear and significant benefits: to essential partnerships, not the much larger number of desirable partnerships at any one time. The risk of partnership overload is real. Senior managers sometimes have to be involved in as many as 60 partnerships (Cairns and Harris 2007). The capacity ceiling is a clear and present constraint. A lack of will is often confused with a sheer lack of capacity – 'we have many more alliance opportunities than we have managers to pursue them. We have to have a way to prioritise' (David Payton, FedEx's managing director of strategic alliances quoted in *Mastering Alliance Strategy*).

Target cultures

With the rise in target cultures in the late 1990s, organisations were given hundreds of new targets, which soon became overwhelming. Ten years later, government policy is to reduce the volume of data collection and processing by 30 per cent, and to reduce the number of targets and performance indicators dramatically, moving to clearer outcome-based national data indicator sets. Progress is slow as dismantling bureaucracy always proves harder than setting it up in the first place, particularly complex electronic data collection systems for which large numbers of staff have been recruited and trained. The tendency in the UK has been to establish ever more complex databases and procedures, especially when a high-profile mistake has been made, but that in turn can lead to key front-line staff spending more time on paperwork and less time on direct work with service users. (Flanagan 2008, in relation to police officers). As the Conservative Party's Commission on Social Workers found, 'One social worker commented that she thought that communication and understanding between professionals was getting worse, particularly as other professions had a lack of understanding of how families interact. She also stated that technology seems to be increasingly seen as 'the answer' to problems with inter-agency work, with core forms driving the assessments rather than the other way round. This often leads to inflexibility as every family is different' (Conservative Party 2007).

An enquirer to the IdEA discussion about partnerships asked 'has anyone done any work around the potential to rationalise strategic partnership arrangements in response to the development of sustainable community strategies and local area agreements? My members and partners are questioning the value of existing structures and overlaps between strategic partnerships such as RAG, Children's Safeguarding Board and LSP and have asked if there are opportunities to re-visit arrangements'. There were no responses (Improvement and Development Agency Website Forum).

Overload comes from several different directions. A special school for 96 blind and partially-sighted children had three separate inspections by the regulator Ofsted in 2006, and had little time to concentrate on anything else. The much-worn but still relevant phrase is 'constantly weighing the pig doesn't make the pig fatter', despite the counter-adage being, 'what is measured gets done' – both are needed in moderation.

People problems

Poor behaviour lies behind many failures in partnership working. At recent Labour Party conferences, 25–30 NHS chief executives assembled to meet a minister or ministers of the day, to hold a frank exchange of views about the NHS. At the conference in Bournemouth in 2007, no minister turned up, and one minister who was in his room at the hotel refused to go down to the meeting, leaving the chief executives seething. Sometimes it's very simple. Twenty-five per cent of hearing impaired people miss their appointments through a lack of communication.

Poor personal behaviour plays a bigger part in partnership collapses than is often realised or admitted. Unchecked power struggles frequently erode partnerships from within. A leader who chairs meetings badly or a key partner who talks endlessly (possession of the mouth) and never lets anyone else get a word in, will switch people off from attending meetings or staying involved, however important the cause. Excessively competitive behaviour or a failure to take any responsibility for a problem is another personal behaviour which makes other partners feel they will bear a disproportionate share of the blame if a mistake is made, rather than a more mature joint responsibility – sharing model evolving through positively managing crises and challenges together.

The nature of the work itself

Stressful work drives front-line care workers inwards, with the risk they shut down and stop looking outwards. At its extreme, this can lead to burnout or even post-traumatic stress disorder, if acutely distressing events have been repeatedly witnessed. 'Care workers who care for traumatised people are particularly vulnerable themselves to secondary trauma' (Cairns and Furnsland 2007). One of my first calls on an emergency duty shift as a young social worker was to a flat where children were inside screaming. When I went in with a police officer, we found two children, by then sobbing, aged five and two. Their mother was lying dead on the floor and their father, who had shot her, had hung himself and was dangling from a ceiling joist – I often wonder how those children are now. Secondary trauma is when the distress of a service user starts to affect the care worker personally, or, as Cattanach wrote about play therapy with abused children:

> helping can also be 'addictive' to the exclusion of everything else. The therapist becomes damaged and such 'addiction' can induce total burnout. The therapist needs to understand the emotional effects of her work on herself and also recognise the wider factors of workplace organisation which can also reinforce the helplessness of the therapist
> (Cattanach 2008)

Social care workers benefit from a range of emotional health and well-being programmes their organisation has a duty to make available to them – through its statutory duty of care. These include risk assessments for staff at risk of secondary trauma; recovery programmes, including formalised peer support or professional companionability during the recovery period; and possibly counselling and a reduced workload for a time-limited period. This is where partnerships within teams come into their own. Most teams will support colleagues to the hilt (Dowling *et al.* 2004). A greater difficulty arises from chronic and endemic low-level stress which is felt by many front-line professionals, and is the 'stress that dare not speak its name'. It is difficult to talk about, difficult to detect, and usually needs treatment of some description, whether that is psychological or pharmacological.

Agency-sponsored support groups can help staff affected by work-related stress, anxiety or depression. The Richard Group was formed in Suffolk

County Council, following the suicide of a social worker in a community mental health team, who was totally committed to his work to a fault. No one was aware of the stress Richard felt, not even his wife and daughters. The Richard Group, supported by Richard's widow and children, holds annual events to honour Richard's contribution and to continue to highlight the issues for a workforce of over 5,000. In a hard hat environment, workers look out for each other.

Avoidance

It is an occasionally unwarranted assumption that everyone involved in a partnership wants it to work. Some agencies, and some individual social care workers, are 'isolationist' and can be described as 'partnership-phobic'. Avoidant families, or 'captive clients' (Thoburn 1980), do everything they can to avoid their social worker, perhaps because they are being assessed for the risks they pose to their children, or because a mental health admission is in prospect. Avoidant or reluctant professionals do everything they can to avoid direct contact with certain service users, either through fear, high stress levels, or cynicism. A percentage of 'no reply' visits can be partly due to professional avoidance, and this can increase the risks to the vulnerable person or people involved. Avoidant partnerships are where key members of the partnership see no point in becoming or staying involved.

The tendency for professional subgroups to bind themselves together through negative comments about people who use their services or their customers was first described by the social scientist Erving Goffman, who talked of what happened 'backstage' (Goffman 1970). A Facebook group which asks bus drivers to share their stories about passengers has comments like 'those slow dim-witted ignoramuses who irritate the hell out of us every day'. As a 16-year-old working on a summer vacation in the gardens of my local crematorium, I first encountered this, when some of the permanent staff would point to smoke coming from the chimneys, making comments like 'death warmed up'. Most professions, including the most prestigious, have the same regrettable trait from time to time – satirising or ridiculing the people who depend on them – and who indirectly pay their salary. The link with partnership culture is when staff in one team or agency organise themselves against a perceived external enemy, putting the shutters up against any new developments. This can of course happen inside an organisation, between front line staff and management for example.

When researching a book on the interface between child protection and adult mental health, one county council I visited in the 1990s had made no progress on service co-ordination because the service managers for child protection and adult mental health respectively could scarcely bear to be in the same room as one another (Douglas and Weir 1999).

Relations between some professional groups and institutions have had such deep fault lines through them for so long, change towards more joined-up working will need a radical fillip. Thirty-two per cent of head teachers found social services were 'not very responsive' to their pupil's needs. Twenty per cent said the same for the police and health workers, although colleges, youth offending teams and drug actions teams fared better (*The Guardian* Education supplement, 8 January 2008). Whilst 90 per cent of head teachers agree they are having 'more of a social services' role as a result of *Every Child Matters*, 56 per cent find this unacceptable. These concerns which at times border on mutual distrust and antipathy have been there throughout my professional career, with daily flashpoints about what information can be shared, and about the status of discussions about individual children.

'Binge' partnerships are a subset of avoidant partnerships. There, organisational behaviour is so manic partnerships are constantly on and off: all the rage for short periods, then ignored for long periods – after pressure to get going subsides.

Lack of clarity about accountability

Lack of clarity about who is responsible for any given service or activity can be a recipe for confusion in partnership working, with dual treble or even quadruple accountabilities at times. The pace of change, including increased complexity, more bureaucratic demands and inexorable scope creep in many projects, has given rise to the metaphor of the 'congested state with its plethora of overlapping jurisdictions, constructed in the name of public benefit but actually confusing the nature of accountability' (Sullivan and Skelcher 2002).

Co-terminosity, where all organisations in a partnership work within the same geographical boundary, makes accountability clearer, but many organisations restructure their organisations without any reference to their partners. Of Scotland's 32 local authorities, only two (Dumfries and Galloway, and Fife) have co-terminous boundaries with their main partners, and Strathclyde Police is a partner in 12 Community Planning Partnerships (CPPs). Lack of clarity can have worse consequences. In parts of London, one side of the street belongs to one London borough and the other side to another, sometimes leading to turf wars about who should take responsibility in an emergency, and slowing response times, despite clear protocols.

Constant change in the NHS over the last decade illustrates many of the dilemmas about accountability. The Department of Health has changed regional and local structures continuously, as well as many of the key operating rules, leaving many health professionals bewildered. By 2002, 303 primary care trusts (PCTs) were set up. At that stage they were not permitted to share management teams and boards. Three years later, a rationalisation process began, cutting the number of PCTs down considerably, as well as reducing the number of strategic health authorities at the regional level – sharing teams and boards was encouraged. The wheel was beginning to turn full circle again, as it often does.

The involvement of the private sector in new developments like Independent Treatment Centres, brought in to provide operations faster and more cost effectively than local hospitals could manage, came at a cost. By 2007, many were only functioning at 70 per cent capacity, and local specialist units in hospital were becoming concerned that they were having to do all the follow up work from these more 'detached' bulk operations. Concerns were also rising that stripping out profitable surgery from NHS hospitals meant it was becoming harder to train the doctors of the future in the core skills they needed because the private sector took no responsibility for the way the medical profession as a whole was developing.

References

Ahgren, B., 2007, 'Creating integrated care: evaluation and management of local care in Sweden', *Journal of Integrated Care*, 15(6): 14–21.

Allnock, D., Tunstill, J., Akhurst, S. and Garbers, C., 2006, 'Constructing and sustaining a Sure Start local programme partnership: lessons for future inter-agency collaborations', *Journal of Children's Services*, 1(3): 29-40.

Anning, A., Cottrell, D., Frost, N., Green, J. and Robinson, M., 2006, *Developing Multi-Professional Teamwork for Integrated Children's Services*, Buckingham: Open University Press.

Atkinson, B.A., *The Atkinson Review: Final Report*, 2005, London: Palgrave. The Atkinson review of the measurement of government output, published by the Office for National Statistics (ONS), 2005, London.

Audit Commission, 1998, *A Fruitful Partnership – Effective Partnership Working*, London: Audit Commission.

Bamford, J., Gomes-Casseres, B. and Robinson, M., 2003, *Mastering Alliance Strategy*, San Francisco: Jossey-Bass.

Bell, D., 2007, interviewed in *Transformation: Promoting New Thinking in the Public Sector*, London: Capgemini and the National School of Government.

Belsky, J., Barnes, J. and Melhuish, E., 2007, *The National Evaluation of Sure Start: Does Area-based Early Intervention Work?*, Bristol: Policy Press.

Bolton, M., 2002, *Voluntary Sector Added Value – a Discussion Paper*, London: NCVO.

Bown, S., 2003, *Scurvy*, Chichester: Summersdale Publishers.

Cairns, B. and Harris, M., 2007, 'Bridge over troubled water? collaboration to improve collaboration across the non-profit/government sector divide', (unpublished paper).

Cairns, K. and Fursland, E., 2007, *Trauma and Recovery: A Training Programme*, London: BAAF.

Carrier, J. and Kendall, I., 1995, *Health and the NHS: Conflict and Change in Britain – A New Audit*, London: Continuum International Publishing Group.

Cattanach, A., 2008, *Play Therapy with Abused Children*, London: Jessica Kingsley.

Chekhov, A., 1991, *The Cherry Orchard*, London: Dover Publications.

Conservative Party, 2007, *No More Blame Game – The Future for Children's Social Workers: Conservative Party Commission on Social Workers*, London: Conservative Party.

CSCI, 2006, *A New Outcomes Framework for the Performance Assessment of Adult Social Care*, London: CSCI.

Douglas, A. and Weir, A., 1999, *Conflict of Interest: Child Protection and Adult Mental Health*, Oxford: Butterworth Heinemann.

Dowling, B., Powell, M. and Glendinning, C., 2004, 'Conceptualising successful partnerships', *Health and Social Care in the Community*, 12(4): 309–17.

Edwards, A., 2007, 'Partnership working and outcomes: the hare and the tortoise?', *Journal of Integrated Care*, 15(1): 24–6.

Fagan, P., Horn, C., Edwards, C., Woods, K. and Caprara, C., 2007, *Outcome Based Evaluations: Faith-based Social Service Organisations and Stewardship*, Washington DC: The Heritage Foundation.

Filkin, G., 2007, 'Better outcomes, better value', in P. Diamond (ed.), *Public Matters*, London: Policy Network.

Flanagan, R., 2008, *The Review of Policing: Final Report*, London: Home Office.

Frost, N., 2005, *Professionalism, Partnership and Joined-up Thinking*, Totnes: Research in Practice, Dartington Hall Trust.

Garrett, L. and Lodge, S., 2008, 'Working together on the front line: how to make multi-professional teams and partnerships work', Totnes: Research in Practice, Dartington Hall Trust.

Glendinning, C., Powell, M. and Rummery, K., 2002, *Partnerships, New Labour and the Governance of Welfare*, Bristol: Policy Press.

Glendinning, C., Halliwell, S., Jacobs, S., Rummery, K. and Tyrer, J., 2000, 'New kinds of care, new kinds of relationships: how purchasing services affects relationships in giving and receiving personal assistance', *Health and Social Care in the Community*, 8(3): 201–11.

Goffman, E., 1970, *Asylums: Essays on the Social Situation of Mental Patients and Other Inmates*, Harmondsworth: Pelican Press.

Hardy, B., Hudson, B. and Waddington, E., 2003, *Assessing Strategic Partnership: The Partnership Assessment Tool*, London: Office of the Deputy Prime Minister.

Hudson, B., 2002, 'Inter-professionality in health and social care: the Achilles heel of partnership?', *Journal of Inter-Professional Care*, 16(1): 7–18.

Hudson, B. and Hardy, B., 2002, 'What is a successful partnership and how can it be measured?, in C. Glendinning, M. Powell and K. Rummery (eds), *Partnerships, New Labour and the Governance of Welfare*, Bristol: Policy Press.

Huxham, C. and Vangen, S., 2005, *Managing to Collaborate*, London: Routledge.

Jordan, B. and Jordan, C., 2000, *Social Work and the Third Way, 'Tough Love as Social Policy'*, London: Sage.

Lasker, R.D., Weiss, E.S. and Miller, R., 2001, 'Partnership synergy: a practical framework for studying and strengthening the collaborative advantage', *The Millbank Quarterly*, 79(2): 179–205.

Markwell, S., 2003, *Partnership Working: A Consumer Guide to Resources*, London: Health Development Agency.

Miller, E., Whoriskey, M. and Cook, A., 2008, 'Outcomes for users and carers in the context of health and social care partnership working: from research to practice', *Journal of Integrated Care*, 16(2): 21–8.

Moran, P., Jacobs, C., Bunn, A. and Bifulco, A., 2007, 'Multi-agency working: implications for an early intervention social work team', *Child and Family Social Work*, 12: 143–51.

Nuffield Institute for Health, 2000, *Assessing Strategic Partnerships: A Partnership Assessment Tool*, Leeds: Nuffield Institute for Health.

Percy-Smith, J., 2006, 'What works in strategic partnerships for children', *Children and Society*, 20: 313–23.

Petch, A., 2007, 'Putting the evidence into performance measurement', *Journal for Integrated Care*, 15(6): 4–5.

Pierson J., 2008, *Going Local*, London: Routledge.

Quinney, A., 2006, *Collaborative Social Work*, Transforming Social Work Practice, Lyme Regis: Learning Matters.

Scott, J., Mannion, R., Davies, H. and Marshall, M., 2003, 'The quantitative measurement of organisational culture in health care: a review of the available instruments', *Health Services Research*, 38(3): 92–95.

Scull, A., 1977, *Decarceration: Community Treatment and the Deviant – A Radical View*, London: Prentice Hall.

Smith, M. and Beazley, M., 2000, 'Progressive regimes, partnerships and the involvement of local communities; A framework for evaluation', *Public Administration*, 78(4): 855–78.

Sullivan, H. and Skelcher, C., 2002, *Working Across Boundaries: Collaboration in Public Services*, Basingstoke: Palgrave.

Thoburn, J., 1980, *Captive Clients: Social Work with Families of Children Home on Trial*, London: Routledge.

West, M. and Markiewicz, L., *The Effective Partnership Working Inventory*, Working Paper, Birmingham: Aston Business School.

8   The future of partnership working

Key messages

- Partnership working has a future, and a strong one
- Demographic trends over the next 25 years will see a rapid rise in demand for services, and continuous pressure on resources means effective partnership working will be crucial to ensure public money and services are better co-ordinated than they are now
- Joint performance management and joint information systems will become standard practice within a decade
- The stories of people whose lives have been transformed by partnership working between themselves and social care professionals should give us heart

---

'Learn to bond, even with your enemy'.
(Kohlrieser 2008)

Scenario planning

In any discussion of the future, it is a mistake to think of the world as a predictable place, as many major trends and events lie outside the realm of normal expectations and are hard to foresee (Taleb 2007). Research on inter-species embryos (or human admixed embryos, or in the tabloid version, human–animal hybrids) is pushing the boundaries of what we might mean by 'a person' in the future. New biofuels and exhaust-free engines make the prospect of environmentally clean cars a realistic prospect. New technology is being developed all the time. For example, hafnium, which is replacing silicon and revolutionising computer chip technology, will double the speed of computing over the next ten years. The 'semantic web', based on much greater data linking and integration, will replace the 'world wide web (www), providing the intelligence to display and analyse trends, compared to the feast of raw data on the current web.

Governments in the UK have positioned themselves as sponsors of partnership and integration, and this is likely to continue at a rapid pace, at the level of superstructure and strategy. In social care, more progress has been made in children's services than adult services which as Cozens says, 'still lacks a unifying concept' (Cozens 2008), although the Law Commission's review of the current hotchpotch of adult social care law may assist. It will need such a unifying vision if government policies such as achieving equality for disabled people by 2025 are to be realised. For practitioners, the massive changes going on above them have never been that visible or that significant, though they can have a steadily sapping impact which is rarely taken seriously by leaders, especially with countervailing power like trade union muscle a shadow of its former self in the 1980s and 1990s. This in itself risks an ever-widening gap between practitioner and managerial cultures, which prompted Kellerman to suggest that focusing on followers and how they can best be motivated to change is just as important as promoting the benefits of strong leadership (Kellerman 2007).

Over the course of a generation, some things change in social care and some don't. Hard drugs on the street are different, more potent, and cheaper, with a bag of heroin costing the same as a bottle of spirits, but the personal and social dynamics for people misusing drugs remain much the same. We know more today: elder abuse was little recognised or understood 20 years ago, whereas it is now acknowledged as a mainstream social problem.

The achievements of social care and its colleague professions have been immense, which gives hope for the future. On current building rates, it will take 55 years to solve London's homelessness problem, but, at the risk of over-simplifying, if homelessness can be eliminated by 2065, a social problem which has scarred lives for centuries will have been solved by sustained and relentless political and social action – and problem-solving partnerships.

Yet just as some problems recede in significance, others increase. The consequences of all-age obesity for health and social care services in the future are unquantifiable, and a direct result of rapidly advancing 'affluenza' (James 2007).

The need to re-conceptualise partnership working, in order to adopt a cross-sectoral framework rather than a parallel perspective, is advocated by Cairns and Harris, who argue that:

> future research could benefit from conceptualising cross-sectoral partnerships not so much as the sum of individual actions in different sectors, and not so much as curious hybrid organisational forms (Evers and Laville, 2004; Minkoff, 2002) but as phenomena which need to be understood as organisational forms in their own right, demanding their own specialist theoretical developments (McDonald, 2005; Milofsky, 2001).
>
> (Cairns and Harris 2007)

Later in this chapter, I propose that a Partnership Institute be established to do just this.

Grounds for optimism about partnership working

Anyone who doubted partnership working is achievable, even in the most unpromising of environments, need look no further than the first power sharing government in Northern Ireland, in which the Rev. Ian Paisley is First Minister and Martin McGuinness is Deputy First Minister. Fifteen years ago, few thought peace would be possible this side of 2020, so bitter was the political, religious and emotional divide. Yet a poll in August 2007, conducted for the *Belfast Evening Telegraph*, found that 67 per cent of a cross-section of people in Northern Ireland felt Paisley and McGuiness were working together 'very well or quite well', compared with 24 per cent six months previously (source: Opinion poll carried out for the *Belfast Evening Telegraph* between 15 June and 11 July 2007, published on 9 August 2007).

The collective realisation that no side could win outright victory over the other led to Paisley and McGuinness's decision to work together. The fact that both of them were branded as extremist pariahs by the British government, and felt themselves to be outsiders, also showed how much they had in common. The role of other politicians in Northern Ireland like David Trimble and John Hume, who spent decades seeking to bridge the gap between Nationalist and Unionist communities whilst Paisley and McGuiness were venting rhetorical hell and fury upon each other, is less well publicised, but equally significant. Even in the most intense conflicts, behind-the-scenes dialogue takes place aimed at identifying common ground. Deals based on compromise agreements are often floated privately at the same time as being denied publicly. The Peace Process Team of civil servants, based in the Northern Ireland Office, won the prestigious, 'winner of winners' Cabinet Secretary's Award in the *Whitehall and Westminster World* Civil Service Awards 2007, for being what Senator George Mitchell, US envoy to Northern Ireland and chairman of the all-party talks, called:

> a class act; energetic, creative and highly skilled professionals. They believed passionately in what they were trying to achieve and they showed the leadership, drive and sheer determination to achieve it.
>
> (quoted in *Whitehall and Westminster World*, November 2007)

The key issue in partnership working is to maintain communication, otherwise months or years can drift by with no contact at all between individuals or agencies who should be working together.

Self-interest and mutual interest are usually aligned in a successful partnership. Partnerships can be like a forced marriage, an arranged marriage or a relationship based on consent. Where a partnership is forced or arranged, it is less likely to be successful than if teams or agencies decide of their own accord to work together by consent, but even that is not a guarantee of success. Partly due to mounting public expectation, which the politicians concerned realised would find its way into votes at future elections, the US delegation at the Bali Climate Change talks agreed for the first time to adopt a plan to negotiate a global warming pact between all nations by 2009 – interests were becoming more aligned.

To date, no such over-riding driver is 'out there' in the social care world, to make partnership working the incontrovertible choice for agencies and professionals on the ground, despite it becoming the first choice for policy makers, and despite the countless Trimbles and Humes at work throughout social care and its partner professions. As discussed in Chapter 5, the tougher technical hurdles to get over before a merged organisation can get off the ground are a counsel of caution. These are arguments in favour of combining services without combining structures.

Partnership working models developed in health and social care are being increasingly adopted by other government agencies. The Borders Agency has introduced a case ownership model for certain categories of immigration case. Its Chief Executive, Lin Homer, says 'we can learn a lot from social work and the dangers of not following cases through' (*Public* magazine, September 2007). A person with learning disabilities is co-director of service development at the Department of Health. By 2007, there were in the region of 5,500 public sector partnerships in the UK, responsible for £5 billion of public expenditure (Audit Commission figures). In every corner of the UK, small local partnerships are in place for hundreds and thousands of services, literally helping millions of people. Built upon commitment and goodwill, this unassuming army of mostly volunteer-led and professionally supported services are the true heart of social care partnerships. In a small town in Cornwall, a woman started up a unisex dance group and, as a direct result, youth crime fell dramatically (Children and Young People Now Awards 2007).

Much of what is provided in the UK is world-class. When the English Minister for Children, Beverley Hughes, spoke to an audience of child care professionals in New York in 2007 about the level of early years provision in the UK, they were amazed at how much we provide. Several UK models such as assertive outreach services have many applications across the social care spectrum, and, whatever the difficulties, are part of a growing suite of community-based practice models that open up the possibility of eventually being able to leave the era of institutional care behind forever. This would have been the promised land for reformers a quarter of a century ago, and it will happen in most of our lifetimes. Compare that achievement in social care with the still rising prison population and the programme to build huge new Titan prisons, in another part of the public sector, where 96 per cent of criminal justice expenditure goes on what has already happened, and only 4 per cent on what to do next.

Grounds for caution: the resources challenge

Ironically, at a time when lifelong support needs have been legally recognised for the first time, in areas such as adoption support services, we are beginning to realise as a society just how much care vulnerable people need and how expensive it is. Unfortunately, this awareness does not extend to a permissive attitude to increasing taxes to pay for that care.

The demographic time bomb throughout the UK is that older people's social care costs (in England) are predicted to rise from £10.1 billion in 2002 to £24 billion in 2026 (at 2005 prices), a gap much wider than private or social insurance policies are likely to bridge, even with big anticipated rises in premiums and contributions that we are already beginning to see. The rise also threatens Scotland's much proclaimed policy of free personal care, introduced in 2002 but so popular by 2008 that it faced a £40 million funding shortfall (Sutherland 2008). Care home costs are predicted to double within the next 20 years (Saga Group 2008). The number of unpaid family carers is expected to rise from 6 million to 9 million by 2037, with a potential shortfall of 2 million (source: Carers UK). Support for people with long-term conditions will require an ever-greater share of social care budgets (see below). Underlying under-funding was estimated at £2 billion a year. (Wanless 2006).

Following his review of health and social care in Wales, Wanless proposed a partnership model for England, based on a formula for splitting personal care costs for people over 65 between the state and the individual (Wanless 2003,

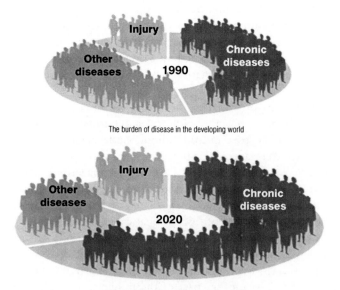

Figure 8.1 The burden of disease in the developing world (Source: Ellis 2008)

2006) Other key changes which are likely to be introduced by 2020 include national entitlement criteria for social care, perhaps financed more through the tax and benefits system than through local authorities. The over-85 population in the UK is expected to double to more than 1.8 million by 2028, and at present half the people over 85 receive a care package of some description from the state. Other statistical projections are worrying, such as the projection of 3.5 million depressed older people and 1 million older people with dementia by 2021. A pandemic of depression in later life is forecast, just as previous generations faced pandemics of cholera and typhoid (see Figure 8.1 for the scale of the increase in long-term conditions).

Even allowing for probable improvements in effective drug treatment, these demographic changes and resource constraints will place a huge added burden on informal carers, more than on state services, which can only spend up to their cash limits.

Informal carers do not have such a cash limit, and changes in personal and family lifestyles may have consequences for the numbers of informal carers available to bridge the 'care gap'. Despite government policy being to provide universal care services, the numbers of children and adults in need but outside the criteria for the provision of state services is set to increase inexorably year on year (CSCI 2008a).

It is important to be as precise as possible about future trends, to avoid prematurely alarmist scenarios. For example the number of unaccompanied asylum-seeking children in England has fallen from 12,000 in 2001 to around 8,500 in 2005, although they do make up an increasing proportion of looked-after children, up from 2 per cent in 2001 to 5.5 per cent in 2007, from 1,500 to 3,300 (source: DCSF figures). The number of suicides is showing a slight decline over the last few years. Whilst stillbirths in the UK are declining, they are increasing in Scotland. The interpretation of trends is notoriously difficult, but it is all that policy makers and planners have.

The importance of key demographics to good scenario planning can be illustrated in the projection of the number of senior public sector staff due to retire between 2010 and 2014. Half of school headteachers will be retiring within the next six years (source: National College of School Leadership), and a similar figure holds true across the public sector. The average age of local councillors in England is 57.8; 70 per cent are men and only 3.5 per cent are from ethnic minority communities (IdeA 2004). Too few leadership development programmes are in place, especially for black and ethnic minority communities, to prepare the political and professional leaders of the future.

Having said that, the profile of social workers is being raised through a sustained government emphasis on the recruitment and retention of social workers. This is based on the successful programme to improve teacher recruitment and retention which started in 1995, six years before the programme for social workers. From 2003, there were more applicants than places on social work qualifying courses for the first time for several years. Having said that, academic thresholds onto social work courses are not on a par with other professions and both vacancies and turnover for children's social workers in English local authorities stood at 9.6 per cent – compared to a 0.6 per cent vacancy rate for teachers (source: DCSF figures, 2008).

Service development trends: implications for partnership working

Whilst services are being delivered through broader and more inclusive partnership structures like new trusts and 'trust arrangements' (Care, Health and Social Care, Children's Foundation), service delivery itself is becoming more specialist, in recognition of the complexity of cases and the knowledge base needed to respond to that need most effectively. An example is the growth of specialist courts in some American states, to replace local courts which deal with every civil criminal or family problem, in a 'McJustice' model (Judge the Honourable Leonard Edwards, founder of the American FDAC, in a speech marking the opening of the first specialist family Drug and Alcohol Court in the UK). So there are drink-driving courts and domestic violence courts, run by specialist judges, a trend unlikely to be picked up wholesale in the UK due to a lack of resources.

Although work with vulnerable people will continue to take place primarily on a face-to-face basis, the internet has a huge potential to reach isolated and vulnerable people who find face to face help hard to accept, however much they are 'reached out' to. A new Norwich-based project called Beat (Beating eating disorders), gets 2 million hits on its website every month (www.b-eat.co.uk). In the UK, 1.1 million people are affected by an eating disorder, and they have the highest mortality rate of any psychiatric illness. Beat presented a survey report, *Something's Got to Change*, to parliamentarians showing only one per cent of sufferers could speak to their parents about their illness. Many service providers report that men in particular prefer web-based to face-to-face communication, and for busy people, a web-based facilitated self-assessment service can enable them to access services they might otherwise reject.

This has been called 'the self-directed services revolution' (Leadbetter, *et al.* 2008), in which a 'somersault effect' is created, standing a traditional service on its head to form a new one. Part of this revolution has been driven by the internet. A particular challenge for web-based service development is to cater for people who use services for whom English is not a first language.

Social care, as happened with social work before it, continues to develop radical social policies. For example, adoption events allow approved adopters to meet and mix with a group of children whose care plan is for adoption, to promote placement chemistry. It is a controversial practice, but one that in the future may find families for some of the 1,500 children and young people still on the Adoption Register at any one time in England and Wales, who are legally freed for adoption but for whom adoption agencies have not been able to find a family. An adoption party in Massachusetts was attended by 92 children in 2007, with many times that number of potential parents.

A Partnership Institute

A Partnership Institute could organise all knowledge about partnership working across government, through a partnership between a lead government department, a university, working with a broad alliance of private and voluntary sector organisations. It should not be confined or led by social care, but should embrace all partnership activity across government, and across the public, private and not for profit sectors. Specialist agencies, academic centres and partnership professionals should be key associate members, and the institute should develop an electronic library and web service to its members. This would be of value to all sectors. For example, at the time of writing, the Royal Bank of Scotland had 850 members in its shared services teams, working in partnership with internal and external customers. It is likely that up to five million staff across all sectors would be able to draw on a properly organised knowledge service about partnership working. The Institute could also store and make available knowledge from a range of areas where there is a growing expectation about working in partnership, such as interfaith programmes, and forgotten partnerships such as that between soldiers and their animals during the history of warfare ('The Animals' War', exhibition at the Imperial War Museum North, Manchester, 2007). In this sense, a Partnership Institute could make a civilising contribution to public life.

What do we now know about partnership working?

I hope I have been able to convey something of the knowledge base for partnership working that now exists. Good social care practice has always been with us, and now has a better chance of success due to the level of knowledge available about what works. Similarly, bad practice has always been with us and shows no sign of being eradicated. Partnership working makes a significant contribution to good practice just as poor inter-agency working is nearly always a feature of bad practice. This knowledge does need to be brought together in one place. In my view, this could be in a high-profile partnership institute. Partnership working is mainstream, yet there is no partnership sector that has emerged from the last 15 years of development. The danger is that, without a central body, there is a constant re-invention of partnership strategies and models, as if it is always being attempted for the first time – organisations without memories acting out a professional Groundhog Day (Ramis 2002). It would help if knowledge about partnership working could be brought together in an accessible place and format.

Policy development

Clearer priorities and joint performance management

Particularly in Chapter 5, I set out the main ways in which a successful social care partnership can be developed. However, legislative support for partnership working remains weak, with few enforceable 'duties of partnership', despite more duties to co-operate appearing on the statute books of UK countries. Performance management regimes still force agencies to meet their own targets, sometimes at the expense of other partners, or in isolation from them. Joint performance management systems remain rare, though they are now starting to increase.

Partnership working needs a set of parallel drivers on the ground, to put flesh on a legislative skeleton. This also requires a reconceptualisation, or a set of policy shifts. For example, considering parental mental health and child welfare, Stanley suggests that 'parental mental health needs to be conceptualised as a response to parenting under adversity – shifting the service menu, and that the preventive value of mental health input in the perinatal period is acknowledged by increasing access to mental health services for families (Stanley 2008).

Clearer priorities for service providers are needed. At the moment, everything is a priority, and the urgent is rarely distinguished from the important. Every new report or plan has new priorities for all concerned to start working on, usually before existing priorities are delivered. Clearer priority-setting and a shared performance management framework are badly needed throughout the public sector.

It is early days. Many new partnerships are only just starting out and only just beginning to think of joint statements of purpose, shared objectives and outcome-based joint targets. The quickest way to establish partnership working would be to make all public service organisations set out a joint statement of purpose with their key partners; to publish joint targets; to publish a joint self-assessment of how the partnership is developing and delivering, which the relevant external inspectorate(s) then quality assure(s); and to develop a joint service user feedback system to ensure people receiving services are satisfied. To do this effectively requires further evolution of the current performance regime aimed at single agencies, even though that raises questions about the accountability of the individual organisation for its core business, and how that is measured and audited. However, some rebalancing of the performance management and funding regime towards both requiring and incentivising partnership working is essential.

Caution about future mergers

Despite the lack of evaluation of recent mergers in the public sector, more are planned. For example, the General Register Office and the Passport Office merged in April 2008, at the same time as some current merger plans are being shelved and some are being disbanded soon after starting up, such as the Assets Recovery Agency (ARA), launched in 2003, whose powers will be transferred to the Serious Organised Crime Agency (SOCA). High costs and misplaced strategy are the usual reasons for an immediate overhaul.

One purpose of a merger is to consolidate similar services and activities in one organisation, for reasons set out in Chapter 5. A good example of a simplification and unification measure has been the unified rights-based mental health and capacity legislation in Northern Ireland following the Bamford Review, leading to a single framework for all people who have decisions taken on their behalf (Bamford 2007).

For other de-mergers or mergers, the logic of government policy is often lost on those most closely involved. Talking about the abolition in 2008 of the Commission for Public and Patient Involvement in Health (CPPIH), the outgoing chief executive said, 'I think it was a clash of government priorities, like the left and the right hand not knowing what they're doing to be honest. It's like, 'we need to reduce our arms-length bodies by half, this is a new one and hasn't been established yet, so we might as well axe it' (Dr Steven Lowden, quoted in *Whitehall and Westminster World*, 15 January 2008).

Similarly, Sir Ian Kennedy, Chair of the Health Care Commission, criticised the proposed merger between CSCI, the Health Care Commission and the Mental Health Act Commission into the Care Quality Commission because he foresaw his inspectors being distracted by two years of upheaval, with the risk they might take their eyes off the ball (*The Guardian*, 9 January 2008). Concerns continue about whether the new commission will lose its social care and indeed its specialist mental health focus.

Health and social care 'raise distinct policy issues' (CSCI 2008b), and with such a massive regulatory span, 'If something goes wrong at St Thomas's Hospital, and something goes wrong at "The Laurels" down Acacia Avenue, which is going to get the attention? I am afraid the National Health Service hospitals will get the attention' (Cumberlege 2008).

The importance of detailed independent oversight of all health and social care service is illustrated by the Commission's investigation into the impact of the superbug *C. difficile* on patients in Maidstone Hospital, run by Maidstone and Tunbridge Wells NHS Trust. The report into events stated

> The Trust told us there were no deaths that were definitely caused by *C. difficile* between April 2004 and March 2006. In the Health Care Commission's sample of 50 patients who had died and had contracted *C. difficile*, our experts found that in 26% of cases, *C. difficile* had definitely or probably contributed to the patient's deaths ... [and] ... A particularly distressing practice reported to us was of nurses telling patients sometimes to 'go in the bed', presumably because this was less time-consuming than helping a patient to the bathroom. Some patients were left, sometimes for hours, in wet or soiled sheets, putting them at

increased risk of pressure sores ... The Trust had no effective system for surveillance of *C. difficile*. As a consequence it failed to identify an outbreak in 2005 that involved 150 patients.

(Health Care Commission 2007)

Public, professional and political confidence

A key reason to change and improve public services is the need to increase public confidence, and to combat the erosion of what used to be a much higher level of trust in professional groups. Unfortunately, this may not benefit social workers, who have always held a feared, and sometimes hated, status in the public mind because of their powers to remove people of all ages from their homes against their will – in some children's computer games, the appearance of a social worker is a 'game-over' moment (Conservative Party Commission on Social Workers 2007). Confidence is higher amongst people who actually use services than those who discuss them without any direct experience, whose views can be influenced by negative media coverage, admittedly of appalling cases where social care staff have made serious and undeniable mistakes. The case of Victoria Climbié is one such. It left a nation puzzled, about how such a shocking set of events could have happened. Victoria's family and friends too remain shattered. 'Up to this day, I still can't get my head around it', said Patrick Cameron, who babysat Victoria, at a public event organised by the Victoria Climbié Foundation in 2006. As Grace Quansah, one of Victoria's cousins said, 'Nobody bothered to talk to Victoria'.

As McLaughlin says:

> Alongside the development of a more democratised welfare state, greater public scepticism about science and expert knowledge has meant that the knowledge base of many professional practices in social work, health and social care has been questioned. This has been evident around issues as diverse as the removal, retention and use of human organs and tissue; vaccination; embryology; adoption, fostering and child protection policies; and 'community care'.

(Maclaughlin 2006)

Trust now has to be earned case by case.

Expectations of social care, and all public services are rightly high, and often too high to meet. A survey by the Caring Choices Coalition, comprising fifteen major charities in the field, found that 34 per cent of people believed public funding should be available for people with low support needs – whereas invariably it isn't (Caring Choices 2008).

Public confidence can be increased by powerful advocates speaking out on issues and speaking up for vulnerable people. The appointment of a Welsh

Commissioner for Older People, building on the Children's Commissioners in all four UK countries, means that issues affecting older people in Wales can be given a higher profile, even if the most influential advocates cannot necessarily dictate to the government of the day. Shortly before he died, the first Welsh Commissioner for Children told me, not entirely tongue in cheek, that his major achievement had been to secure improvements in the state of the toilets in schools in the former Glamorgan local authority areas.

The duty to co-operate – should it have more teeth?

We saw in Chapter 2 how an increasing number of duties to co-operate are being placed on statutory organisations, usually accompanied by guidance that emphasises partnerships have to be inclusive, particularly to guard against risks of excluding third sector organisations and representatives of people who use services. For example, from April 2008, an early years outcomes duty was placed on local authorities by the Childcare Act 2006, to work with the NHS and Jobcentre Plus 'to improve the five *Every Child Matters* outcomes of all young children in their area and reduce inequalities between them, through integrated early childhood services'. These days, Jobcentre Plus have childcare partnership managers in each of their districts – the product of ever-rising expenditure on partnership posts across the public sector.

As we have also seen, legislation on its own has limited impact. It can create new enabling powers and duties, and it can set targets to measure how they are being implemented. However, it is locally that the partnership will produce the intended outcomes, if it going to at all, so the answer to,'should legislation have more teeth?' is no. It is the way in which the duty to work together in partnership is interpreted that makes the difference.

We have already seen that having the right structures, systems, strategies and plans is important, but that this does not guarantee that progress will be made. Many strategies are written because they have to be, without there ever being a serious intention to do anything about them. We have also seen that new duties tend to be placed on the same managers and practitioners responsible for dealing with existing initiatives, limiting the time they have to devote to any single partnership development. We have also seen how local partnership cultures, personalities and practicalities, are often the reason why a partnership gels.

As Frost says in his research review of efforts to integrate children's services, 'the most effective joined-up working emerges from actual practice' (Frost 2005). Whilst research is limited, it bears this out. For example, in a study of 256 older people at risk of care home entry, which compared assessments by care managers with assessments by care managers and geriatricians jointly, the joint assessments, through identifying covert morbidity, led to joint service provision which enabled a lower rate of entry to nursing homes, improved outcomes for users and carers, and lower costs of care (Challis *et al.* 2004).

Whilst expectations about the duty to co-operate can be made clear by politicians, and whilst systems such as co-located services and clear operational protocols can be put in place by managers, good partnership outcomes can only be achieved by front-line practitioners working well together.

Is there such a phenomenon as a partnership gene, to be cultivated?

Partnership working is evolving, with some long-life partnerships surviving, even as the bulk of partnerships to date have been short-life for all the reasons I have described. If there is a trend, it is towards looser networks and coalitions on specific issues and services, rather than grandiose all-encompassing trusts, even if 'trusts' exist in name and statute. The trend towards smaller and more locally relevant and responsive services, increasingly shared with and defined by people who use services themselves, fits with this. In the search for a defining partnership model, 'the quest will be for a citizen-based model of integration' (Integrated Care Network 2008).

Where larger organisations have taken over smaller organisations, in a classic imitation of private equity behaviour, in which the best of the smaller organisation is retained, and the worst sacrificed, there is as yet little sense of new better hybrid operational cultures emerging as a result. In the case of some of the larger merged organisations which are diversifying, and looking to enter the health and social care market through new services like polyclinics, there is no evidence as yet that they can bring the full resources of the private firm or corporation to transform a public service. No, the partnership gene, if there is one, is not especially transformational – it is just everyday social care people reproducing themselves.

In social care partnerships today, when you want to change the way a service works or operates, you should not look for the right person – you should look for the right alliance. Contemporary service provision and government is not an arena for superheroes. It needs clever and committed people who can work together using a team approach to make steady progress towards solving perennially difficult strategic and operational problems, and for those individuals to demonstrate good partnership working in case after case and situation after situation.

Story telling

I want to end by telling the stories of some more individuals, as social care is in the final analysis about helping individual people overcome profound disadvantage. Marla Runyan is a successful blind distance runner who can't see the finish line. The singer Ayo was born in 1980. Her mum was a heroin addict, her dad kidnapped her from a foster home, and she was moved between many foster homes, yet her music is powerful and reaches out to others (*Joyful*, 2007, Polydor Records).

Early in 2008, I met a group of young people in the English care system, who were talking about their lives. I could have had the same conversation with them when I started out in social work, 33 years ago. The reasons they were in care were the same as then. Several had parents no longer able to care for them due to persistent and enduring mental health problems. Some had been abandoned by their parents whilst living with them, and they in turn had rejected their parents, with the wounds still open. Some were isolated, despite being in care for years, including one 15-year-old boy who had lived in 64 placements, most of them like brief, functional hotel nights. One young person asked why she had no choice of foster carer before being sent to a new placement, raising the same question about having a choice being raised by adults with disabilities who need and use social care services. One young woman had been pushed at 16 to live independently, years before she was ready. Some had real ambitions and hope for themselves, despite their unpromising start in life, whilst some were close to despair and seemingly heading towards the infamous revolving door of adult institutions in a few year's time. Each child or young person had more people around her or him than when I started out. Indeed, several talked about how confusing it was to have so many people to relate to – most wanted just one and for that one person to be more consistent and readily available. In the end, individual stories and accounts tell you more than anything else about the real state of play in partnership working. Those stories, of heartbreak, despair and hope, need to be heard and acted upon, again and again, as if they are being heard for the first time.

Conclusion

The partnership obligation

Any in-depth look at a single social care case, or discussion with a vulnerable service user who quickly reveals multiple needs, many that can't be met, shows how essential it is that service users, their carers and professional agencies have to work together to provide the best service possible in what are invariably tough and difficult circumstances. Partnership working is best viewed as an obligation – the partnership obligation. Any message that working together is optional rather than mandatory leaves too many vulnerable people in difficulty or at risk.

The improvement in the quality of life stemming from a simple set of partnerships can be a reason in itself to continue with it, as Glenys's story below demonstrates. Hers is a partnership with a housing provider and a support worker, and many others behind the scenes. To be able to answer your own front door and say yes or no to who comes in, rather than living residentially and having no control over who comes and sits next to you, is one positive outcome to celebrate, for Glenys and for the social care profession. To be able to make a cup of tea when you want it, not at a set

Glenys's story

I've lived in a residential care home in Lancashire for seven years and before that I lived with my parents who, as much as I dearly love them, wrapped me up in cotton wool. I have no front door key or control over who supports me or how they do it. I am going to be moving into my own flat in Fleetwood. I will have my own front door key and there will be a shared lounge when I can spend time with my neighbours whenever I like. I will receive an independent budget to spend on my support. I will interview staff who work with me and spend part of it on support round the home to help me with domestic tasks like cooking my own meals and managing my money as I've never done it by myself before. I will use my budget of £14,000 a year to employ someone to support me at college where I will go on a computer course. I also want to do voluntary work. I also hope to pool some money with my neighbours to employ a craft teacher. I want to learn to swim and will spend money on someone to help me into the pool. I also want to go into Manchester as I haven't seen it since it has been rebuilt. I will also pay for a friend to go on holiday with me so she can support me there.

All these things will be included in my support plan which I will review with Kate in three months. I'll know it is working if I am doing all the things I have talked about such as voluntary work. I feel for the first time in 61 years that I am in control of my own life and it is a great feeling.

Source: speech by Glenys Fisher at a GSCC Parliamentary reception on the personalisation of care services, 22 April 2008

time, is equally liberating. The central purpose of partnership working is to improve the quality of life for each and every social care user.

We will get there!

Social care has never been able to define itself clearly as a separate professional discipline and as a vital public service held in high long-term regard. It has recently been merged structurally with the NHS and education to be part of a broader set of integrated services. Despite the risks of it always playing second fiddle, this gives partnership working an ever-stronger statutory framework. The steady fruit of the push on partnership working can be illustrated by the virtual disappearance of major tensions between the NHS and local councils overdelayed transfers of care of older people from hospitals to community settings. These tensions reached boiling point in the years between 2000 and 2005, culminating in legislation to introduce a system of fines that could be levied on local authorities for what was colloquially – and pejoratively – known as 'bed blocking'. By 2008, few figures were collected nationally any longer about this, and the numbers of cases causing concern had dramatically reduced. New partnership programmes such as all-inclusive intermediate care services had made a significant difference.

Similarly, when I co-authored a book on the interface between child protection and adult mental health in 1999, few organisations integrated both services. However, by 2008, the Family Welfare Association's (FWA) Building Bridges service had 12 branches across England, offering a range of family support services and interventions to provide exactly that integrated service.

Progress on the ground is evident in enough areas to contemplate a time when partnership working will eventually become redundant terminology because it is a way of life, even if, to paraphrase the little girl from a primary school (see page 5) I can do partnership working ... but not yet.

A few years ago, I asked an audience of 400 city brokers and hedge fund managers attending a charity function, how many of them had adopted a child, were adopted or knew a close relative or friend with an adopted child. Over half of this random audience put up their hands. We know from research how common mental illness is in the general population, and how common, for example, is caring for a relative with disabilities. When I collected my CBE from the Queen in February 2008, I stood with a rear-admiral, the Chief of Staff to the Second Sea Lord, who happened to be receiving the same award. His *Who's Who* entry states that he spends considerable time 'developing coping strategies for a close relative with Asperger's Syndrome'. Most people in the UK are personally connected to social care issues or services at some stage in their lives. In that sense if in no other, it is a universal service, and because of the nature of the problems it deals with, a universal partnership service. Long may it remain as such.

References

Bamford, D., 2007, *Equal Lives: Review of Policy and Services For People with a Learning Disability in Northern Ireland* (The Bamford Report), Belfast: Reivew of Mental Health and Learning Disability (NI).

Cairns, B. and Harris, M., 2007, 'Bridge over troubled water? Collaboration to improve collaboration across the non profit/government sector divide', (unpublished paper).

Caring Choices Coalition, 2008, *The Future of Care Funding: Time for a Change*, London: Caring Choices Coalition.

Challis, D., Clarkson, P., Williamson, J., Hughes, J., Venables, D., Burns, A. and Weinberg, A., 2004, The value of specialist clinical assessments of older people prior to entry to care homes, *Age and Ageing*, 33(1): 25–34.

CSCI (Commission for Social Care Inspection), 2008a, *The State of Social Care in England*, London: CSCI.

CSCI (Commission for Social Care Inspection), 2008b, *Grand Committee Brief on the Health and Social Care Bill – Part 1*, London: CSCI.

Conservative Party Commission on Social Workers, 2007, *No Blame Game*, London: Conservative Party.

Cozens, A., 2008, 'Poor Law care due for an upgrade', *The Guardian* Society supplement, 6 February.

Cumberlege, J., 2008, Debate on the Health and Social Care Bill, 21 April, House of Lords.

Ellis, T., 'Long-term conditions whole system demonstrators (WSD)', London: Department of Health.

Evers, A. and Laville, J.L. (eds), 2004, *The Third Sector in Europe*, Cheltenham: Edward Elgar.

Frost, N., 2005, *Professionalism, Partnership and Joined-up Thinking*, Totnes: Research in Practice, Dartington Hall Trust.

Health Care Commission, 2007, *Investigation Into outbreaks of* Clostridium difficile *at Maidstone and Tunbridge Wells NHS Trust*, London: Health Care Commission.

IdeA and Employers Association for Local Government, 2006, *National Census of Local Authority Councillors*, London: IdeA.

IdeA, 2007, *Making it Real: A Report of the Pilot Partnership Improvement Programme with Voluntary and Community Organisations and Local Authorities*, London: IdeA.

Integrated Care Network, 2008, *A Practical Guide to Integrated Working, 2008*, Leeds: Care Services Improvement Partnership.

James, O., 2007, *Affluenza*, London: Vermilion.

Kellerman, B., 2007, 'What every leader needs to know about followers', *Harvard Business Review*, December: 84–91.

Kohlrieser, G., 2008 *The Hostage at the Table*, San Francisco: Josey-Bass.

Leadbetter, C., Bartlett, J. and Gallagher, N., 2008, *Making it Personal*, London: Demos.

McDonald, I., 2005, 'Theorising partnerships: governance, communicative action and sport policy', *Journal of Social Policy*, 34(4): 579–600.

McLaughlin, E., 2006, 'Pseudo-democracy and spurious precision: knowledge dilemmas in the new welfare state', in C. Glendinning and P. Kemp (eds), *Cash and Care*, Bristol: Policy Press.

Milofsky, C., 2001, 'Intermediate structures: expanding knowledge about nonprofit transorganisations', paper presented to the annual meeting of the Association for Research on Nonprofit Organisations and Voluntary Action (ARNOVA), Miami, Florida.

Minkoff, D., 2002, 'The emergence of hybrid organisational forms: combining identity-based service provision and political action', *Nonprofit and Voluntary Sector Quarterly*, 31(3) 377–401.

Ramis, H., 2002, *Groundhog Day*, Sony Pictures Home Entertainment.

Saga Group, 2008, press release, 'Final cost of long-term care to double in 20 years', www.saga.co.uk.

Stanley, N., 2008, *Children's and Adults' Services: Interagency Communication*, London: Parental Mental Health and Child Welfare Network in partnership with the Social Perspectives Network.

Sutherland, S., 2008, *Independent Review of Free Residential and Nursing Care in Scotland*, Edinburgh: Scottish Government Publications.

Taleb, N.N., 2007, *The Black Swan*, Harmondsworth: Penguin.

Wanless, D., 2003, *The Review of Health and Social Care in Wales*, Cardiff: Welsh Assembly.

Wanless, D., 2006, *Securing Good Care for Older People: Taking a Long-Term View*, London: Kings Fund.

Index

Lightning Source UK Ltd.
Milton Keynes UK
UKOW04f0245170514

231796UK00006B/36/P